PLANS OF CARE FOR
SPECIALTY PRACTICE

Ambulatory Pediatric Nursing

PLANS OF CARE FOR
SPECIALTY PRACTICE

Ambulatory Pediatric Nursing

MEG GULANICK, PhD, RN
Assistant Professor
Niehoff School of Nursing
Loyola University of Chicago
Chicago, Illinois

MICHELE KNOLL PUZAS, MHPE, RNC
Pediatric Nurse Clinician
Michael Reese Hospital and Medical Center
Chicago, Illinois

DEIDRA GRADISHAR, BS, RNC
Obstetric Outreach Educator
University of Chicago Perinatal Network
Assistant Clinical Manager, Birth Rooms
University of Chicago Hospitals
Chicago, Illinois

KATHY V. GETTRUST, RN, BSN ~ *Series Editor*
Case Manager
Midwest Medical Home Care
Milwaukee, Wisconsin

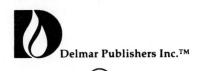

Delmar Publishers Inc.™

I(T)P™

NOTICE TO THE READER

Publisher does not warrant or guarantee any of the products described herein or perform any independent analysis in connection with any of the product information contained herein. Publisher does not assume, and expressly disclaims, any obligation to obtain and include information other than that provided to it by the manufacturer.

The reader is expressly warned to consider and adopt all safety precautions that might be indicated by the activities described herein and to avoid all potential hazards. By following the instructions contained herein, the reader willingly assumes all risks in connection with such instructions.

The publisher makes no representations or warranties of any kind, including but not limited to, the warranties of fitness for particular purpose or merchantability, nor are any such representations implied with respect to the material set forth herein, and the publisher takes no responsibility with respect to such material. The publisher shall not be liable for any special, consequential or exemplary damages resulting, in whole or in part, from the readers' use of, or reliance upon, this material.

Delmar publishing team:
Publisher: David C. Gordon
Administrative Editor: Patricia Casey
Associate Editor: Elisabeth F. Williams
Project Editor: Danya M. Plotsky
Production Coordinator: Mary Ellen Black
Art and Design Coordinator: Megan K. DeSantis
                             Timothy J. Conners

For information, address

Delmar Publishers Inc.
3 Columbia Circle, Box 15015
Albany, NY 12212-5015

Printed in the United States of America
Published simultaneously in Canada
by Nelson Canada,
a division of The Thomson Corporation

1   2   3   4   5   6   7   8   9   10   XXX   00   99   98   97   96   95   94

Library of Congress Cataloging-in-Publication Data

Gulanick, Meg
    Ambulatory pediatric nursing / Meg Gulanick, Michele Knoll Puzas, Deidra Gradishar.
      p.   cm.—(Plans of care for specialty practice)
    Includes bibliographical references and index.
    ISBN 0-8273-5256-5
    1. Pediatric nursing.   2. Ambulatory medical care for children.   3. Nursing care plans.   I. Puzas, Michele Knoll.   II. Gradishar, Deidra.   III. Title.   IV. Series.
    [DNLM: 1.   Pediatric Nursing.   2. Ambulatory Care—nurses' instruction.   WY159]
RJ245.G85   1994
610.73′62—dc20
DNLM/DLC
for Library of Congress   93-32200
                                                                                              CIP

TABLE OF CONTENTS

HEALTH TEACHING GUIDES

CONTRIBUTORS

JoAnn Allen, RN, BSN
Clinic Nurse, University of Chicago
  Hospitals
Wyler Children's Hospital
Chicago, Illinois
• Sickle Cell Anemia

Barbara Ruth Bellar, PAC
Physicians Assistant, Michael Reese
  Health Plans
Chicago, Illinois
• Conjunctivitis

Renee Bluml, RD, CNSD
Pediatric Nutrition Specialist
Michael Reese Hospital and Medical
  Center
Chicago, Illinois
• Infant Nutrition

Peggy Cowling, RNC, MSN
Clinical Nurse Specialist, Obstetrics/
  Gynecology
South Suburban Hospital
Hazel Crest, Illinois
• Urinary Tract Infection

Susan Geoghegan, RN, BSN
Pediatric Staff Nurse
Michael Reese Hospital and Medical
  Center
Chicago, Illinois
• Anemia

Barb Hartz, RN, MS, CNP
Clinical Nurse Manager
Child and Adolescent Center
Evanston Hospital
Evanston, Illinois
• Pertussis

Kathleen Jaffry, RN
Pediatric Staff Nurse
Michael Reese Hospital and Medical
  Center
Chicago, Illinois
• Diabetes Mellitus
• Pneumonia

Bernadette Keller, RN, BSN
Staff Nurse, Labor and Delivery
Michael Reese Hospital and Medical
  Center
Chicago, Illinois
• Scarlet Fever

Cathleen Kiely, RN, BSN
Pediatric Staff Nurse
Michael Reese Hospital and Medical
  Center
Chicago, Illinois
• Child Abuse/Neglect

Audrey Klopp, RN, PhD, ET
Director, Medical-Surgical Nursing
Michael Reese Hospital and Medical
  Center
Chicago, Illinois
• Crohn's Disease

Daria Lieber, RN
Staff Nurse, Obstetrics/Gynecology
Michael Reese Hospital and Medical
  Center
Chicago, Illinois
• Pinworms

Alison Benzies Miklos, RNC, MSN
Neonatal Clinical Nurse Specialist
  Outreach Educator
Christ Hospital and Medical Center
Perinatal Center
Oak Lawn, Illinois
• Colic
• Safety
• Sleep
• Teething

Lillian Navarrete, RN
Pediatric Staff Nurse
Michael Reese Hospital and Medical
  Center
Chicago, Illinois
• Diarrhea
• Fever

Ellen Polite, RN
Pediatric Staff Nurse
Michael Reese Hospital and Medical
  Center
Chicago, Illinois
• Measles, German (Rubella)
• Mumps (Parotitis)

Michele Knoll Puzas, RNC, MHPE
Pediatric Nurse Clinician
Michael Reese Hospital and Medical
  Center
Chicago, Illinois
• Asthma
• Cast Care
• Chicken Pox (Varicella)
• Hemophilia
• Immunizations
• Infant Nutrition
• Lead Poisoning
• Measles (Rubeola)
• Otitis Media
• Pediculosis Capitis (Head Lice)

Caroline Reich, RN, MS
Nurse Manager, Obstetrics, Nursery
  and SCN
Riverside Hospital
Kankakee, Illinois
• Circumcision Care
• Diaper Rash (Diaper Dermatitis)

Dawn E. Reimann, RN, MS
Outreach Educator
Rush-Presbyterian-St. Lukes
Perinatal Center
Chicago, Illinois
• Colic
• Safety
• Sleep
• Teething

Carol Reman, RN, MSN, PNP
Certified Pediatric Nurse Practitioner
Child and Adolescent Center
Evanston Hospital
Evanston, Illinois
• Candidiasis

Sandra N. Roberts, RN, MSN
Instructor
St. Xavier University
Chicago, Illinois
• Idiopathic Thrombocytopenic
  Purpura

Kathleen Scharer, RN, MS, CS,
  FAAN
Clinical Nurse Specialist, Psychiatry
Lutheran General Hospital
Park Ridge, Illinois
• Attention Deficit Disorder
• Dysfunctional Grieving
• Substance Abuse

Ruth Novitt Schumacher, RN, MSN
Instructor, Maternal Child Health
University of Illinois at Chicago
Chicago, Illinois
• Impetigo
• Pharyngitis

Nedra Skale, RN, MS, CNA
Nurse Clinician, Department of
  Surgery
Division of Pediatric Surgery
Michael Reese Hospital and Medical
  Center
Chicago, Illinois
- Abdominal Pain, Acute
- Abdominal Pain, Persistent or
  Recurrent
- Acne
- Gastroesophageal Reflux/Pyloric
  Stenosis
- Hernia, Inguinal
- Hernia, Umbilical
- Seizures (Febrile)
- Undescended Testicle
  (Cryptorchidism)
- Vomiting

Marlene Smith, RNC, MSN, FNP
Family Nurse Practitioner
Child and Adolescent Center
Evanston Hospital
Evanston, Illinois
- Dental Hygiene: Caries Prevention
- Safety

Diana Stephens, RNC, NP
Outreach Educator
University of Chicago Hospital
Chicago, Illinois
- Bronchopulmonary Dysplasia

Linda Walsh, RN, BSN
Pediatric Staff Nurse
Michael Reese Hospital and Medical
  Center
Chicago, Illinois
- Constipation

Jeffrey Zurlinden, RN, MS
Director
Community Program for Clinical
  Research on AIDS
Chicago, Illinois
- Chlamydia
- Gonorrhea
- Growth and Development
  - First Year
  - Toddler
  - 3–5 Years
  - 6–9 Years
  - 10–12 Years
  - Adolescence
  - Growth Charts
- Herpes
- Syphilis

PREFACE

*A*mbulatory Pediatric Nursing was developed to provide nursing care planning guides to address pediatric issues seen in various ambulatory settings. Developed for the practicing nurse, we envisioned these guides being used by office and clinic nurses, nurse practitioners and emergency room nurses, and any nurse needing a handy reference for planning pediatric patient care. We also believe that this book can be an information source for nurses working in women's health care settings, where questions about child health often are raised.

Utilizing the expertise of 26 contributors, the selected topics range from a section devoted to growth and development, to purely teaching issues, to common complaints and disease. To take advantage of a language familiar to all nurses, the nursing process format and nursing diagnoses were used in a concise, practical application. For the novice and student, rationales are included to explain the complex and assist in decision making.

Although the topic selection is not all inclusive, we believe a wide spectrum is contained herein that includes much that is not frequently addressed elsewhere in this manner. We hope this text can assist you in caring for your pediatric patients and their families.

Meg Gulanick
Michele Knoll Puzas
Deidra Gradishar

ACKNOWLEDGMENTS

Our appreciation to colleagues who have helped with this book:
Barbara Norwitz for her vision and support. The editorial staff, particularly Patricia E. Casey and Elisabeth F. Williams, and the production staff of Delmar Publishers for their expertise and guidance through the publishing process. Roseann O'Malley for her quality work in preparing the manuscript. Our contributors for their willingness to share their expertise. To all our children, who teach and delight.

SERIES INTRODUCTION

Scientific and technological developments over the past several decades have revolutionized health care and care of the sick. These rapid and extensive advancements of knowledge have occurred in all fields, necessitating an ever-increasing specialization of practice. For nurses to be effective and meet the challenge in today's specialty settings, the body of clinical knowledge and skill needs to continually expand. *Plans of Care for Specialty Practice* has been written to aid the practicing nurse in meeting this challenge. The purpose of this series is to provide comprehensive, state-of-the-art plans of care and associated resource information for patient situations most commonly seen within a specialty that will serve as a standard from which care can be individualized. These plans of care are based on the profession's scientific approach to problem solving—the nursing process. Though the books are written primarily as a guide for frontline staff nurses and clinical nurse specialists practicing in specialty settings, they have application for student nurses as well.

DOCUMENTATION OF CARE

The Joint Commission on Accreditation of Healthcare Organizations (JCAHO) assumes authority for evaluating the quality and effectiveness of the practice of nursing. In 1991, the JCAHO developed its first new nursing care standards in more than a decade. One of the changes brought about by these new standards was the elimination of need for every patient to have a handwritten or computer-generated care plan in his or her chart detailing all or most of the care to be provided. The Joint Commission's standard that describes the documentation requirements stipulates that nursing assessments, identification of nursing diagnoses and/or patient care needs, interventions, outcomes of care, and discharge planning be permanently integrated into the clinical record. In other words, the nursing process needs to be documented. A separate care plan is no longer needed; however, planning and implementing care must continue as always, but using whatever form of documentation that has been approved by an institution. *Plans of Care for Specialty Practice* can be easily used with a wide variety of approaches to documentation of care.

ELEMENTS OF THE PLANS OF CARE

The chapter title is the presenting situation, which represents the most commonly seen conditions/disorders treated within the specialty setting. It may be a medical diagnosis (e.g., diabetes mellitus), a syndrome (e.g., acquired immunodeficiency syndrome), a surgical procedure (e.g., mastectomy), or a diagnostic/therapeutic procedure (e.g., thrombolytic therapy).

An opening paragraph provides a definition or concise overview of the presenting situation. It describes the condition and may contain pertinent physiological/psychological bases for the disorder. It is brief and not intended to replace further investigation for comprehensive understanding of the condition.

Etiologies

A listing of causative factors responsible for or contributing to the presenting situation is provided. This may include predisposing diseases, injuries or trauma, surgeries, microorganisms, genetic factors, environmental hazards, drugs, or psychosocial disorders. In presenting situations where no clear causal relationship can be established, current theories regarding the etiology may be included.

Clinical Manifestations

Objective and subjective signs and symptoms which describe the particular presenting situation are included. This information is revealed as a result of a health history and physical assessment and becomes part of the data base.

Clinical/Diagnostic Findings

This component contains possible diagnostic tests and procedures which might be done to determine abnormalities associated with a particular presenting situation. The name of the diagnostic procedure and the usual abnormal findings are listed.

Nursing Diagnosis

The nursing management of the health problem commences with the planning care phase of the nursing process. This includes obtaining a comprehensive history and physical assessment, identification of the nursing diagnoses, expected outcomes, interventions, and discharge planning needs.

Diagnostic labels identified by NANDA through the Tenth National Conference in April 1992 are being used throughout this series. (Based on North American Nursing Diagnosis Association, 1992. *NANDA Nursing Diagnoses: Definitions and Classification 1992*.) We have also identified new diagnoses not yet on the official NANDA list. We endorse NANDA's recommendation for nurses to develop new nursing diagnoses as the need arises and we encourage nurses using this series to do the same.

"Related to" Statements

Related to statements suggest a link or connection to the nursing diagnosis and provide direction for identifying appropriate nursing interventions. They are termed contributing factors, causes, or etiologies. There is frequently more than one related to statement for a given diagnosis. For example, change in job, marital difficulties, and impending surgery may all be "related to" the patient's nursing diagnosis of anxiety.

There is disagreement at present regarding inclusion of pathophysiological/medical diagnoses in the list of related to statements. Frequently, a medical diagnosis does not provide adequate direction for nursing care. For example, the nursing diagnosis of chronic pain related to rheumatoid arthritis does not readily suggest specific nursing interventions. It is more useful for the nurse to identify specific causes of the chronic pain such as inflammation, swelling, and fatigue; these in turn suggest more specific interventions. In cases where the medical diagnosis provides the best available information, as occurs with the more medically oriented diagnoses such as decreased cardiac output or impaired gas exchange, the medical terminology is included.

Defining Characteristics

Data collection is frequently the source for identifying defining characteristics, sometimes called signs and symptoms or patient behaviors. These data, both subjective and objective, are organized into meaningful patterns and used to verify the nursing diagnosis. The most commonly seen defining characteristics for a given diagnosis are included and should not be viewed as an all-inclusive listing.

Risk Factors

Nursing diagnoses designated as high risk are supported by risk factors that direct nursing actions to reduce or prevent the problem from developing. Since these nursing diagnoses have not yet occurred, risk factors replace the listing of actual defining characteristics and related to statements.

Patient Outcomes

Patient outcomes, sometimes termed patient goals, are observable behaviors or data which measure changes in the condition of the patient after nursing treatment. They are objective indicators of progress toward prevention of the development of high-risk nursing diagnoses or resolution/modification of actual diagnoses. Like other elements of the plan of care, patient outcome statements are dynamic and must be reviewed and modified periodically as the patient progresses. Assigning realistic "target or evaluation dates" for evaluation of progress toward outcome achievement is crucial. Since there are so many considerations involved in when the outcome could be achieved (e.g., varying lengths of stay, individual patient condition), these plans of care do not include evaluation dates; the date needs to be individualized and assigned using the professional judgment and discretion of the nurse caring for the patient.

Nursing Interventions

Nursing interventions are the treatment options/actions the nurse employs to prevent, modify, or resolve the nursing diagnosis. They are driven by the related to statements and risk factors and are selected based on the outcomes to be achieved. Treatment options should be chosen only if they apply realistically to a specific patient condition. The nurse also needs to determine frequencies for each intervention based on professional judgment and individual patient need.

We have included independent, interdependent, and dependent nursing interventions as they reflect current practice. We have not made a distinction between these kinds of interventions because of institutional differences and increasing independence in nursing practice. The interventions that are interdependent or dependent will require collaboration with other professionals. The nurse will need to determine when this is necessary and take appropriate action. The interventions include assessment, therapeutic, and teaching actions.

Rationales

The rationales provide scientific explanation or theoretical bases for the interventions; interventions can then be selected more intelligently and actions can be tailored to each individual's needs.

The rationales provided may be used as a quick reference for the nurse unfamiliar with the reason for a given intervention and as a tool for patient education. These rationales may include principles, theory, and/or research findings from current literature. The rationales are intended as reference information and, as such, should not be transcribed into the permanent patient record. A rationale is not provided when the intervention is self-explanatory.

Discharge Planning/Continuity of Care

Because stays in acute care hospitals are becoming shorter due to cost containment efforts, patients are frequently discharged still needing care; discharge planning is the process of anticipating and planning for needs after discharge. Effective discharge planning begins with admission and continues with ongoing assessment of the patient and family needs. Included in the discharge planning/continuity of care section are suggestions for follow-up measures, such as skilled nursing care; physical, occupational, speech, or psychiatric therapy; spiritual counseling, social service assistence; follow-up appointments, and equipment/supplies.

References

A listing of references appears at the conclusion of each plan of care or related group of plans. The purpose of the references is to cite specific work used and to specify background information or suggestions for further reading. Citings provided represent the most current nursing theory and/or research bases for inclusion in the plans of care.

A Word About Family

The authors and editors of this series recognize the vital role that family and/or other significant people play in the recovery of a patient. Isolation from the family unit during hospitalization may disrupt self-concept and feelings of security. Family members, or persons involved in the patient's care, must be included in the teaching to ensure that it is appropriate and will be followed. In an effort to constrain the books' size, the patient outcome, nursing intervention, and discharge planning sections usually do not include reference to the family or other significant people; however, the reader can assume that they are to be included along with the patient whenever appropriate.

Any undertaking of the magnitude of this series becomes the concern of many people. I specifically thank all of the very capable nursing specialists who authored or edited the individual books. Their attention to providing state-of-the-art information in a quick, usable form will provide the reader with current reference information for providing excellent patient care.

The editorial staff, particularly Patricia E. Casey and Elisabeth F. Williams, and production people at Delmar Publishers have been outstanding. Their frank criticism, comments, and encouragement have improved the quality of the series.

Finally, but most importantly, I thank my husband, John, and children, Katrina and Allison, for their sacrifices and patience during yet another publishing project.

Kathy V. Gettrust
Series Editor

LIST OF TABLES

Growth and Development

▼

$\mathcal{F}$IRST YEAR

Jeffrey Zurlinden, RN, MS

Infancy (birth to 12 months) is a time of great physical and cognitive growth. The baby's nervous system and other organ systems become more closely regulated and less variable in function than at birth. The primary caregiver and the infant establish a bond and a mutually satisfying relationship that enables the infant to learn to trust.

▼

NURSING DIAGNOSIS: HIGH RISK FOR ALTERED GROWTH AND DEVELOPMENT

Risk Factors
- Prematurity
- Small for gestational age
- Maternal alcohol or illicit drug use
- Maternal neglect or abuse
- Genetic disorders
- Chronic or acute illness
- Trauma
- Separation from primary caregivers
- Hormonal dysfunction
- Birth trauma or hypoxia
- Malnutrition
- Poisonings or environmental exposures
- Lack of stimulation
- Poverty

Patient Outcomes
- Infant's weight and height will fall between the 5th and 95th percentiles on a standardized, gender-specific growth chart (see Growth Charts, pp 39 and 41).
- Infant's head circumference will fall between the 10th and 90th

3

percentiles on a standardized, gender-specific growth chart (see Growth Charts, pp 39 and 41).
- Infant will demonstrate age-appropriate milestones for gross motor, fine motor, language, social-emotional, reflex, and cognitive development.

Nursing Interventions	Rationales
Physical growth At every visit, measure infant's weight, height, and head circumference. Plot the current data on growth charts and compare with previous measurements. Refer if • infant falls outside the 5th and 95th percentiles for height and weight. • infant falls outside the 10th and 90th percentiles for head circumference. • the pattern of growth has changed substantially. • one measurement is in a very different percentile than the other measurements.	Referral may be necessary to determine significance and causative factors of growth disturbance. Care should be taken to incorporate parental size into evaluation of infant growth.
Observe or palpate for emergence of deciduous teeth. • Lower central incisors erupt at 7–8 months. • Upper central incisors erupt at 9–10 months. • Lower lateral incisors erupt at age 11–12 months.	Absence of or severely abnormal dentition after 10 months will adversely affect nutrition and language development.
Developmental At every visit, interview caregiver and observe infant for the presence of developmental milestones.	Absent or severely delayed gross and fine motor development may indicate neurologic deficit. Refer for evaluation if unable to 1. hold head erect by 3 months. 2. sit independently on firm surface. 3. bear most of weight on legs by 10 months.

Nursing Interventions

Gross motor
- birth—moves all limbs with equal ease and range of motion
- 2 months—lifts head up 45 degrees (range 0–3 months)
- 2.5 months—sits with support and holds head up (range 1.5–4.5 months)
- 4 months—rolls over (front to back first) (range 2–5 months)
- 6.5 months—sits without support (range 5–8 months)
- 9.5 months—pulls self to standing (range 6–10 months)
- 10.5 months—walks holding onto furniture (range 7–13 months)
- 13 months—stands well (range 10–14 months)
- 13.5 months—walks well (range 11–18 months)

Fine motor
- 3 months
  - puts hands together (range 1.5–4 months)
  - follows movement by turning head 180 degrees (range 2–4 months)
- 4 months—grasps rattle (range 2.5–4.5 months)
- 4.5 months—reaches for objects (range 3–5 months)
- 6.5 months—moves cube from hand to hand (range 5–7.5 months)
- 9 months—makes thumb-finger grasp (range 7.5–10.5 months)
- 10 months—bangs cubes together when they are held in hands (range 7–12.5 months)
- 12 months—makes pincer grasp (range 9–15 months)

Nursing Interventions

Language
- birth—responds to sounds
- 1 month—babbles or makes sounds other than crying (range 1–2 months)
- 2.5 months—laughs (range 1.5–3.5 months)
- 7.5 months—turns to voice (range 4.8–5 months)
- 9 months—says "mama" or "dada," but indiscriminately (range 6–10 months)
- 9.5 months—imitates speech sounds (range 6–11 months)
- 12.5 months—says "mama" or "dada," to specific people (range 10–14 months)

Social-emotional
- birth—regards face (usually at birth, range 0–1 month)
- 3 months—smiles spontaneously (range 1.5–5 months)
- 6 months—feeds self crackers (range 5–8 months)
- 7 months—plays peek-a-boo (range 5.5–9.5 months)
- 9.75 months—shy with strangers (range 5.5–10 months)
- 10 months—plays pat-a-cake (range 7–13 months)
- 14 months—drinks from a cup (range 10–17 months)

Rationales

Poor or absent social-emotional and language development may indicate neurological disorder or hearing deficit. Refer if
1. no response to voices or common noises by 2 months.
2. doesn't turn to sounds by 6 months.
3. doesn't babble by 10 months.
4. doesn't attend to words by 12 months.
5. hands are not fisted at 4 months.
6. doesn't hold objects in hands by 7 months.
7. unable to chew lumpy foods by 10 months.

Nursing Interventions	Rationales

Reflexes
 Interview the caregiver and elicit the following reflexes from the infant:
 • Moro reflex (present at birth and disappears by age 6 months)
 • asymmetrical tonic neck reflex (may not be present at birth, usually strong by age 2–3 months and disappears by age 6 months)
 • unusual or inappropriate repetitive movements of mouth and tongue
 • feeding difficulties related to sucking, swallowing, or moving food with the tongue
 	
 Cognitive
 • 2–4 months—simple acts are repeated and gradually become intentional as they have the desired effect on the object
 • 5–8 months
   – infant develops a rhythm of eating, sleeping, and eliminating in synchrony with caregiver
   – infant gradually increases expression of needs, crying, reaching
 • 8–12 months—goal-directed behaviors present, infant searches, imitates	

Nursing Interventions

Play
1. Ask the caregiver about the infant's play activities.
2. Suggest appropriate toys (avoid toys with lead paint or other toxic surfaces, or with pieces small enough to swallow).
   - newborns enjoy: black/white shapes, parents' faces
   - 0–3 months enjoys: nursery mobiles, stuffed toys, gentle rocking and carriage rides, music boxes
   - 4–6 months enjoys: bright toys small enough to grasp, squeeze toys, bouncing on adult's lap or knee, splashing in the bathtub
   - 7–9 months enjoys: pat-a-cake, crawling and rolling over on floor, peek-a-boo, noise makers, busy boxes with movable toys
   - 10–12 months enjoys: push-pull toys, teething toys, take-apart toys, nested boxes, playing ball

Rationales

Toys should be selected with the infant's development in mind—if too complex, infant will not benefit and may disassociate.

▼

NURSING DIAGNOSIS: HIGH RISK FOR KNOWLEDGE DEFICIT (CAREGIVER) CONCERNING EXPECTED GROWTH AND DEVELOPMENT

Risk Factors
- Caregiver is inexperienced with the growth and development of infants.
- Caregiver uses illicit drugs or alcohol to excess.
- Caregiver neglects or abuses child.

Patient Outcomes
Primary caregivers will verbalize
- expected developmental milestones for the infant's current age.
- developmental milestones to expect for the next level of development.

Nursing Interventions	Rationales
Observe interaction between infant and caregivers.	Interactions may demonstrate caregiver's lack of knowledge or other problem.
Ask caregivers what they expect the infant to be doing now and in the near future.	Caregiver may voice expectations inconsistent with infant's age/development.
Demonstrate proper handling of the infant.	
Outline for caregivers the current stage of growth and development and the milestones to expect next.	
Explore the caregiver's concerns, especially feeding, walking, talking, toilet training, and spoiling the infant.	
Review ways to make the home safe for an infant.	Most injuries during the first year of life are preventable (see Safety, p. 287).

▼

DISCHARGE PLANNING/CONTINUITY OF CARE

- Arrange referrals as needed
  - social work
  - self-help groups
  - physical therapy/occupational therapy
  - speech/hearing
  - dietitian
  - family therapy
  - further medical evaluation
- Follow up every 2–3 months during first year.

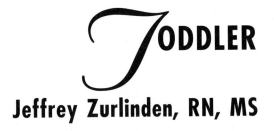

ʗODDLER

Jeffrey Zurlinden, RN, MS

The toddler (12–30 months) asserts his/her own personality by walking and running independently and by talking. Organ systems become more closely regulated and predictable.

▼

NURSING DIAGNOSIS: HIGH RISK FOR ALTERED GROWTH AND DEVELOPMENT

Risk Factors
- Prematurity
- Small for gestational age
- Maternal alcohol or illicit drug use during pregnancy
- Maternal neglect or abuse during pregnancy
- Genetic disorders
- Chronic or acute illness
- Trauma
- Separation from primary caregivers
- Hormonal dysfunction
- Birth trauma or hypoxia
- Malnutrition
- Poisonings or environmental exposures
- Lack of stimulation
- Poverty

Patient Outcomes
- Toddler's weight and height will fall between two standard deviations on a standardized graph (see Growth Charts, pp 39 and 41).
- Toddler's head circumference will fall between the 10th and the 90th percentiles on a standardized, gender-specific growth chart (see Growth Charts, pp 39 and 41).

- Toddler will demonstrate age-appropriate milestones for gross motor, fine motor, language, social-emotional, and cognitive development.

Nursing Interventions

Physical growth
At every visit, measure toddler's weight, height, and head circumference. Refer if
1. toddler falls outside the 5th and 95th percentiles for height and weight.
2. toddler falls outside the 10th and 90th percentiles of head circumference.
3. the pattern of growth has changed substantially.
4. one measurement is in a very different percentile than the other measurements.

Observe or palpate for emergence of deciduous teeth.
1. Lower lateral incisors erupt at 12–13 months.
2. Upper and lower first bicuspids erupt at 15–16 months.
3. Upper and lower cuspids erupt at age 18–19 months.
4. Upper and lower second bicuspids erupt at age 26–27 months.

Developmental
At every visit, interview caregiver and observe child for the presence of developmental milestones.

Rationales

Lack of growth or sudden arrest may indicate illness or social/psychological problem that requires further investigation/treatment. Parents' size/heritage must be considered when comparing child to growth standards.

Lack of motor development may indicate neurological deficit, musculoskeletal or psychosocial problem. Early intervention is beneficial for children with permanent disorders. Refer if unable to
1. walk alone by 18 months.
2. kick when standing by 21 months.
3. release held objects by 15 months.

Nursing Interventions	Rationales

Gross motor
1. Observe that the toddler moves all limbs with equal ease and range of motion.
  • 18 months
    – runs poorly with frequent falls
    – walks backward
  • 24 months
    – throws ball overhand
    – walks up and down stairs
    – kicks ball forward
  • 30 months
    – jumps in place
    – balances briefly on one foot
    – begins to walk on tiptoes
 	
Fine motor
  • 18 months
    – builds a tower with two cubes
    – scribbles spontaneously
  • 24 months
    – builds a tower of four cubes
    – turns doorknobs and unscrews lids
    – turns pages one at a time
  • 30 months
    – builds a tower of eight cubes
    – holds crayons with fingers like an adult	

Nursing Interventions

Rationales

Language
- 18 months
  - understands much more than is able to say
  - vocabulary of about 10 words
  - can identify common objects by pointing
  - may say "no" to mean either "yes" or "no"
- 24 months
  - uses 2–3-word phrases
  - vocabulary of about 300 words
  - likes to talk
  - states basic needs
- 30 months
  - uses plurals
  - follows simple directions

Lack of development may indicate hearing, neurological, or psychosocial deficit. Refer if unable to
1. say single words with proper meaning by 21 months.
2. make 2–3-word phrases by 21 months.

Social-emotional
- 18 months
  - uses spoon with little spilling
  - uses cup with little spilling
  - removes clothes
  - expresses anger by temper tantrums
  - tolerates separation from mother
- 24 months
  - removes shoes
  - helps with dressing
  - plays alongside other children
- 30 months
  - separates from mother more easily
  - plays interactive games
  - knows gender differences
  - fewer tantrums

Toddlerhood is stressful for both child and parent as a result of the struggle between dependence and independence. Lack of socioemotional and cognitive development can be caused by physical/neurological disorders as well as the absence or limitation of cognitive, social and emotional stimulation.

Nursing Interventions	**Rationales**
Reflexes 1. Observe for the persistence of infantile reflexes. 2. Observe the mouth and tongue for unusual or inappropriately repetitive movements. 3. Ask the caregiver about feeding difficulties related to sucking, swallowing, or moving food with the tongue.	
Cognitive 1. Egocentric thinking 2. Begins to recognize that objects continue to exist even when they are no longer seen 3. Begins to learn cause and effect	
Play 1. Ask the caregiver about the play activities. 2. Suggest appropriate toys (avoid toys with lead paint or other toxic surfaces, or with pieces small enough to swallow). 3. Toddlers enjoy: push-pull toys, sandbox, Play-Doh, puzzles, bathtub toys, finger paints, low playground equipment, toy household objects.	Play is considered the work of children. Development and learning are inherent in play; toys and activities should be geared toward individual toddler's abilities.

▼

NURSING DIAGNOSIS: HIGH RISK FOR KNOWLEDGE DEFICIT (CAREGIVER) CONCERNING EXPECTED GROWTH AND DEVELOPMENT

Risk Factors
- Caregiver inexperienced with the growth and development of toddlers.
- Caregiver uses illicit drugs or alcohol to excess.
- Caregiver abuses or neglects child.

Patient Outcomes
Primary caregiver will verbalize
- expected developmental milestones for the toddler's current age.
- developmental milestones to expect for the next level of development.

Nursing Interventions	Rationales
Observe interaction between toddler and caregivers.	
Ask caregivers what they expect the toddler to be doing now and in the near future.	Abuse sometimes stems from child's inability to perform according to caregiver's expectations.
Demonstrate proper handling of the toddler.	
Outline for caregivers the current stage of growth and development and the milestones to expect next.	
Explore the caregiver's concerns, especially toilet training, adjustment to preschool, and discipline.	Parents may have concerns related to the toddler's growing independence and may need parenting suggestions appropriate to toddler's level of development (limit setting, parental approval, praise, allowing choice).
Review ways to make the home safe for a toddler.	

▼

DISCHARGE PLANNING/CONTINUITY OF CARE

- Arrange referrals as needed
  - social work
  - self-help groups
  - family therapy
  - further medical evaluation
- Follow up annually or more often as necessary.

3–5 YEARS

Jeffrey Zurlinden, RN, MS

Because of greater gross motor and fine motor control, and expanding language abilities, the preschooler (3–5 years) learns how to behave as a social person. The child learns a place in the family, makes friends outside of the family, and learns how to behave away from home.

▼

NURSING DIAGNOSIS: HIGH RISK FOR ALTERED GROWTH AND DEVELOPMENT

Risk Factors
- Maternal alcohol or illicit drug use during pregnancy
- Maternal neglect or abuse during pregnancy
- Genetic disorders
- Chronic or acute illness
- Trauma
- Separation from primary caregivers
- Hormonal dysfunction
- Birth trauma or hypoxia
- Malnutrition
- Poisonings or environmental exposures
- Lack of stimulation
- Poverty

Patient Outcomes
- Child's weight and height will fall between two standard deviations on a standardized, gender-specific growth chart (see Growth Charts, pp 40–42).
- Child's head circumference will fall between the 10th and the 90th percentiles on a standardized, gender-specific growth chart (see Growth Charts, pp 40 and 42).

- Child will demonstrate age-appropriate milestones for gross motor, fine motor, language, social-emotional, and cognitive development.
- Primary caregivers will verbalize developmental milestones to expect for the next level of development.

Nursing Interventions	Rationales
Physical growth At every visit, measure the child's weight, height, and head circumference. Plot the current data on growth charts and compare with previous measurements. Refer if 1. child falls outside the 5th and 95th percentiles for height and weight. 2. child falls outside the 10th and 90th percentiles for head circumference. 3. the pattern of growth has changed substantially. 4. one measurement is in a very different percentile than the other measurements.	Growth disturbances must be investigated for significance and causative factors. Cultural patterns of growth must be considered.
Developmental At every visit, interview caregiver and observe child for the presence of developmental milestones.	

Nursing Interventions	**Rationales**

Gross motor
Observe that the child moves all limbs with equal ease and range of motion.
• 3 years
  – peddles tricycle
  – walks up stairs by alternating feet
  – balances on one foot for at least 1 second
  – broad jumps
• 4 years
  – hops on one foot
  – skips
  – walks down stairs by alternating feet
• 5 years
  – skips and hops by alternating feet
  – catches bouncing ball well
    – jumps rope
 	
Fine Motor
• 3 years
  – builds tower of eight cubes
  – can draw a copy of a circle
  – uses a fork held in a fist
• 4 years
  – draws person with three parts
  – uses scissors
  – uses fork held with fingers.
• 5 years
  – ties shoe laces
  – draws person with six parts
  – uses simple tools, pencils, or crayons very well
	Disturbance in motor skills development may indicate a significant neurological/musculoskeletal disorder. Refer if unable to
	1. stand on one foot by 3 years.
	2. hop on one foot by 4 years.
	3. jump rope by 5 years.

Nursing Interventions

Language
- 3 years
  - uses 3–4 word sentences.
  - vocabulary of about 900 words
  - asks questions using "who," "what," and "where"
  - uses plurals and pronouns
- 4 years
  - uses 4–5-word sentences
  - vocabulary of about 1500 words
  - enjoys telling stories
  - uses prepositions
- 5 years
  - uses 6–8-word sentences
  - vocabulary of about 2100 words

Social-emotional
- 3 years
  - able to share toys and play with others
  - usually stays dry throughout the night
  - boys urinate standing
  - able to seat self on toilet
  - dresses with supervision.
- 4 years
  - plays cooperatively with a group of children
  - dresses without supervision
  - independent with toileting
  - mood swings and rebellious behavior
- 5 years
  - helps with household tasks
  - enjoys competitive games
  - uses social manners

Reflexes
Observe for the persistence of infantile reflexes.

Rationales

Lack of development can indicate a hearing deficit or speech or learning disorder. Refer if
1. unable to speak in sentences or speech is unintelligible by 3 years.
2. speech is not fully intelligible by 4 years.
3. stuttering or stammering, or word endings that indicate plurals or tenses are missing by 5 years.

Lack of socioemotional, and cognitive development may indicate a physical disorder or problems in the home/environment. Refer if not toilet trained by 5 years.

Nursing Interventions	Rationales

Cognitive
• 3 years
  – knows first and last name
  – is egocentric
  – differentiates time into past, present, and future
• 4 years
  – recognizes colors
  – counts correctly, but doesn't understand the concept of numbers
• 5 years—thought remains intuitive and egocentric, influenced by what the child wants and how events relate to him/her	

Play 1. Ask the caregiver about the child's play activities. 2. Suggest appropriate toys and activities. 3. A 3–5-year-old enjoys: physical activities, such as running, jumping, climbing, and low slides and swings; storytelling and imaginative fantasy with dolls, people, or animal figures; building and putting together toys with many small pieces; coloring, cutting, and pasting.	Parents may need help in understanding child's needs, especially those that enhance development.

▼

NURSING DIAGNOSIS: HIGH RISK FOR KNOWLEDGE DEFICIT (CAREGIVER) CONCERNING EXPECTED GROWTH AND DEVELOPMENT

Risk Factors
• Caregiver inexperienced with the growth and development of children.
• Caregiver uses illicit drugs or alcohol to excess.
• Caregiver abuses or neglects child.

Patient Outcomes
Primary caregivers will verbalize
• expected developmental milestones for the child's current age.
• developmental milestones to expect for the next level of development.

Nursing Interventions	Rationales
Observe interaction between child and caregivers.	As the preschoolers vocabulary and language skills expand, *questions* become a primary method for learning and socializing.
Ask caregivers what they expect the child to be doing now and in the near future.	
Demonstrate age-appropriate interactions with the child.	
Outline for caregivers the current stage of growth and development and the milestones to expect next.	
Explore caregiver's concerns, especially adjustment to school and safety away from home.	
Review safety measures at home and in the neighborhood.	As the 3–5-year-old develops, he/she becomes more independent and more social. Safety in the neighborhood, such as avoiding streets, pools, strangers, and the like, must be explained to the child with rationales.

▼

DISCHARGE PLANNING/CONTINUITY OF CARE

- Arrange referrals as needed
  - social work
  - family therapy
  - further medical evaluation
- Follow up annually or more often when needed.

6–9 YEARS

Jeffrey Zurlinden, RN, MS

The child of 6–9 years interacts in a wider world that now includes school. He/she is industrious and works hard to master new skills.

▼

NURSING DIAGNOSIS: HIGH RISK FOR ALTERED GROWTH AND DEVELOPMENT

Risk Factors
- Maternal alcohol or illicit drug use during pregnancy
- Maternal neglect or abuse during pregnancy
- Genetic disorders
- Chronic or acute illness
- Trauma
- Separation from primary caregivers
- Hormonal dysfunction
- Birth trauma or hypoxia
- Malnutrition
- Poisonings or environmental exposures
- Lack of stimulation
- Poverty

Patient Outcomes
- Child's weight and height will fall between the 5th and 95th percentiles on a standardized graph (see Growth Charts, pp 40 and 42).
- Child will demonstrate age-appropriate milestones for gross motor, fine motor, language, social-emotional, and cognitive development.

Nursing Interventions

Physical growth

At every visit, measure the child's weight, height, and head circumference. Plot the current data on growth charts and compare with previous measurements. Refer if

- child falls outside the 5th and 95th percentiles for height and weight.
- child falls outside the 10th and 90th percentiles for head circumference.
- the pattern of growth has changed substantially.
- one measurement is in a very different percentile than the other measurements.

Observe for loss of deciduous teeth and eruption of permanent teeth.

- Lower central incisors replaced at 6 years.
- Upper and lower first molars erupt during the sixth year.
- Upper central and lower incisors replaced at 7 years.
- Upper lateral incisors replaced at 8 years.
- Lower cuspids replaced at 9 years.

Developmental

At every visit, interview caregiver and observe child for the presence of developmental milestones

Gross motor

Observe that the child

- moves all limbs with equal ease and range of motion.
- learns to ride bicycle.
- learns to swim.
- loves to run, skip, and jump.
- is still more enthusiastic than coordinated.

Rationales

Altered growth patterns should be investigated for significance and cause.

Significant delay in motor development should be investigated. Some clumsiness is a normal phenomenon.

Nursing Interventions	Rationales
Fine Motor 1. Eye-hand coordination is not yet fully developed. 2. Child is impatient and easily frustrated with activities requiring fine motor skills.	
Language Assess vocabulary and reading level. • Examples of words understood by 75% of 4th-grade students: bulldog, camper, cigar, crocodile, distance, dizzy, dodge, locket, sheriff, sniff, tangle, thirst, widow, weedy, wives. • Children of this age are able to make simple analogies.	Refer for speech therapy if sounds are distorted or omitted, speech is confused, or voice is monotonous, too loud, or too soft.
Social-emotional 1. Ask about friendships at school or in the neighborhood. 2. A 6–9-year-old • needs supervision bathing. • selects clothing for individual reasons.	School and same-sex peers become increasingly important in this age group. There may be difficulty integrating family values with those in the larger world.
Reflexes Observe for the persistence of infantile reflexes.	
Cognitive 1. Ask about school achievement. 2. A 6–9-year-old • knows days of the week. • knows seasons. • is very concrete in thinking. • is detail oriented.	

Nursing Interventions	Rationales
Play 1. Ask about the child's favorite play activities. 2. Suggest appropriate toys, games, and activities. 3. A 6–9-year-old enjoys: making collections, active and rough-and-tumble games, easy board and card games, comic books, trucks, building things, dolls, reading, bicycling, swimming, skateboarding, and rollerblading.	

▼

NURSING DIAGNOSIS: HIGH RISK FOR KNOWLEDGE DEFICIT (CAREGIVER) CONCERNING EXPECTED GROWTH AND DEVELOPMENT

Risk Factors
- Caregiver is inexperienced with the growth and development of children.
- Caregiver uses illicit drugs or alcohol to excess.
- Caregiver abuses or neglects child.

Patient Outcomes
Primary caregivers will verbalize
- expected developmental milestones for the child's current age.
- developmental milestones to expect for the next level of development.

Nursing Interventions	Rationales
Observe interaction between child and caregivers.	
Ask caregivers what they expect the child to be doing now and in the near future.	
Demonstrate age-appropriate interactions with the child.	
Outline for caregivers the current stage of growth and development and the milestones to expect next.	

Nursing Interventions	Rationales
Explore the caregiver's concerns, especially adjustment to school and discipline.	Parents may need help to understand child's need for peer support and allegiance as well as continued parental guidance.
Review safety away from home and when swimming or riding skateboard, bicycle, or rollerblades.	

▼

DISCHARGE PLANNING/CONTINUITY OF CARE

- Arrange referrals as needed
    - dietitian
    - social work
    - speech
    - physical therapy/occupational therapy
    - family therapy
- Follow up annually or more often as needed.

10–12 YEARS

Jeffrey Zurlinden, RN, MS

The child of 10–12 years develops independence in the world outside of the home, makes strong friendships, and highly values the opinions of his/her peer group. Beginning puberty creates emotional and physical turmoil.

▼

NURSING DIAGNOSIS: HIGH RISK FOR ALTERED GROWTH AND DEVELOPMENT

Risk Factors
- Child's alcohol or illicit drug use
- Parental alcohol or illicit drug use
- Maternal neglect or abuse during pregnancy
- Genetic disorders
- Chronic or acute illness
- Trauma
- Separation from primary caregivers
- Hormonal dysfunction
- Birth trauma or hypoxia
- Malnutrition
- Poisonings or environmental exposures
- Poverty

Patient Outcomes
- Child's weight and height will fall between the 5th and 95th percentiles on a standardized graph (see Growth Charts, pp 40 and 42).
- Child will demonstrate age-appropriate milestones for gross motor, fine motor, language, social-emotional, and cognitive development.

Nursing Interventions	Rationales
Physical growth At every visit, measure the child's weight, height, and head circumference. Plot the current data on growth charts and compare with previous measurements. Refer if • child falls outside the 5th and 95th percentiles for height and weight. • the pattern of growth has changed substantially. • one measurement is in a very different percentile than the other measurements.	Altered growth paterns, especially precocious puberty or significantly delayed prepubertal changes, should be investigated for significance and cause.
Observe for loss of deciduous teeth and eruption of permanent teeth. • Upper and lower first bicuspids and upper second bicuspids replaced at 10 years. • Upper cuspids and lower second bicuspids replaced at 11 years. • Upper and lower second molars erupt during 12th year.	
Developmental Assess for achievement of developmental milestones:	

Gross motor
1. Observe that the child moves all limbs with equal ease and range of motion.
2. A 10–12-year-old
  • has greater strength, stamina, and coordination than earlier.
  • enjoys refining favorite skills and talents.
  • is capable of complicated skills that require timing and judgement.
	Lack of motor development may indicate significant musculoskeletal/neurological disorder.

Nursing Interventions

Fine motor
A 10–12-year-old has
- fully developed eye-hand coordination.
- greater patience with activities requiring fine motor skills.

Language
Assess vocabulary and reading level.
- Examples of words understood by 75% of 6th-grade students: adhesive, alto, appetite, bacteria, berth, bridal, campus, davenport, fatherless, fishery, gadget, grit, midst, pardon.

Social-emotional
1. Ask about friendships at school or in the neighborhood.
2. A 10–12-year-old
   - is independent in bathing.
   - has growing awareness of fashion and grooming.

Reflexes
Observe for the persistence of infantile reflexes.

Cognitive
1. Ask about school achievement.
2. A 10–12-year-old
   - is able to perform arithmetic.
   - remains concrete in thinking.

Rationales

Refer for speech therapy if sounds are distorted or omitted, speech is confused, or voice is monotonous, too loud, or too soft.

School and peers remain significant in the child's socioemotional and cognitive development. Difficulties must be investigated before becoming overwhelming to child and destructive to development (see Attention Deficit Disorder).

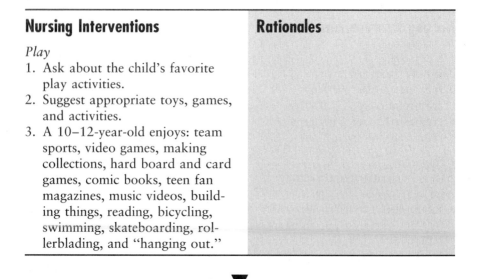

Nursing Interventions	Rationales
Play	
1. Ask about the child's favorite play activities.	
2. Suggest appropriate toys, games, and activities.	
3. A 10–12-year-old enjoys: team sports, video games, making collections, hard board and card games, comic books, teen fan magazines, music videos, building things, reading, bicycling, swimming, skateboarding, rollerblading, and "hanging out."	

NURSING DIAGNOSIS: HIGH RISK FOR KNOWLEDGE DEFICIT (CAREGIVER) CONCERNING EXPECTED GROWTH AND DEVELOPMENT

Risk Factors
- Caregiver is inexperienced with the growth and development of children.
- Caregiver uses illicit drugs or alcohol to excess.
- Caregiver abuses or neglects child.

Patient Outcomes
Primary caregivers will verbalize
- the expected developmental milestones for the child's current age.
- developmental milestones to expect for the next level of development.

Nursing Interventions	Rationales
Observe interaction between child and caregivers.	
Ask caregivers what they expect the child to be doing now and in the near future.	
Demonstrate age-appropriate interactions with the child.	
Outline for caregivers the current stage of growth and development and the milestones to expect next.	

Nursing Interventions	Rationales
Explore the caregiver's concerns, especially sexual development, recreational drug and alcohol use, fiscal responsibility, and discipline.	Parents may need help in addressing issues with child, in allowing progressive independence, and in dealing with outside threats to the child's safety.
Review safety away from home and when swimming or riding skateboard, bicycle, or rollerblades.	

▼

DISCHARGE PLANNING/CONTINUITY OF CARE

- Arrange referrals as needed
  - dietitian
  - social work
  - speech/hearing
  - further medical evaluation
- Follow up annually or more often as needed.

*A*DOLESCENCE

Jeffrey Zurlinden, RN, MS

Each adolescent (13–19 years) searches for his/her unique identity. The opinions of peers remain important, but the adolescent begins to recognize other options. He/she explores sexuality and begins to make truly intimate relationships that may or may not include sex.

▼

NURSING DIAGNOSIS: HIGH RISK FOR ALTERED GROWTH AND DEVELOPMENT

Risk Factors
- Child's alcohol or illicit drug use
- Parental alcohol or illicit drug use
- Neglect or abuse
- Genetic disorders
- Chronic or acute illness
- Trauma
- Separation from primary caregivers
- Hormonal dysfunction
- Birth trauma or hypoxia
- Malnutrition
- Poverty

Patient Outcomes
- Adolescent's weight and height will fall between the 5th and 95th percentiles on a standardized, gender-specific growth chart (see Growth Charts, pp 40 and 42).
- Adolescent will demonstrate development of secondary sexual characteristics.
- Adolescent will demonstrate age-appropriate milestones for gross motor, fine motor, language, social-emotional, and cognitive development.

Nursing Interventions

Physical growth
At every visit, measure the adolescent's weight and height. Plot the current data on growth charts and compare with previous measurements. Refer if
- adolescent falls outside the 5th and 95th percentiles for height and weight.
- the pattern of growth has changed substantially.
- one measurement is in a very different percentile than the other measurements.

Observe for emergence of permanent teeth.
1. Upper and lower third molars erupt between ages 17 and 21 years.

Observe or question the patient about development of puberty.
1. Obtain a menstrual history for girls.
2. Discuss expected development.

Rationales

Significant weight loss may indicate an eating disorder such as bulimia or anorexia nervosa, which could be life threatening.

Early or late, or what may seem early or late, development can be emotionally stressful.
1. Menarche usually begins between ages 10 and 15 years. Age 12.5 is the most common, usually about 2 years after the beginning of breast and pubic hair development. Menstruation is irregular and may not indicate ovulation until 12–24 months after menarche. Development is divided into five stages depending on the growth of the breasts and the distribution of pubic hair.
2. Boys reach puberty between ages 12.5 and 16.5 years. Age 14 is the most common. Development is divided into five stages depending on the enlargement of the penis and testes and the distribution of pubic hair.

Nursing Interventions	**Rationales**
Developmental Assess for achievement of developmental milestones.	
Gross motor 1. Observe that the adolescent moves all limbs with equal ease and range of motion. • Rapid growth during early adolescence may decrease coordination.	Lack of development or decline should be investigated for significance and cause (e.g., muscular dystrophy).
Fine motor Observe for difficulty writing.	

Language
Assess vocabulary and reading level.
• Examples of words understood by 75% of students in
  – 8th grade: amend, archeology, byway, dimension, fluorescent, horoscope, inefficient, laughingstock, lingerie, officialdom, salutation
  – 10th grade: circumstantial, deface, diversion, enshrine, gallows, hinder, implication, negligent, orthodox, pollination, proton, refrain
  – 12th grade: acetylene, aft, buxom, condone, curfew, fascism, heresy, indicative, opportune, oppression, prophetic, secretariat	

Nursing Interventions

Social-emotional
1. Ask about friendships at school or in the neighborhood.
2. Obtain sexual history.
   - If sexually active, obtain specimens for pregnancy test or cultures for sexually transmitted diseases (STDs).
   - Assess level of understanding of birth control and transmission of human immunodeficiency virus, hepatitis B virus, and other STDs.
3. Obtain history of recreational drug and alcohol use.

Reflexes
Observe for the persistence of infantile reflexes.

Cognitive
1. Ask about school achievement.
2. An adolescent
   - begins to understand abstract statements and possibilities.
   - can predict outcomes based on laws or principles.
   - can evaluate an argument in terms of internal logic or consistency.
   - begins to evaluate own behavior, motives, and thoughts.

Play
1. Ask about favorite activities.
2. An adolescent
   - shows greater individuality in recreational activities.
     - What is done may be less important than with whom.
   - enjoys: playing or being a spectator of team sports, video games, music, dancing, movies, bicycling, skateboarding, rollerblading, joy riding, and "hanging out."

Rationales

Social-emotional development in the adolescent is as turbulent for the child and parent as was toddlerhood, but with added threats to safety and health involved as the adolescent again struggles with issues of dependence and independence.

▼

NURSING DIAGNOSIS: HIGH RISK FOR KNOWLEDGE DEFICIT (CAREGIVER) CONCERNING EXPECTED GROWTH AND DEVELOPMENT

Risk Factors
- Caregiver is inexperienced with the growth and development of adolescents.
- Caregiver uses illicit drugs or alcohol to excess.
- Caregiver abuses or neglects adolescent.

Patient Outcomes
Primary caregivers will verbalize the expected developmental milestones for the adolescent.

Nursing Interventions	Rationales
Observe interaction between adolescent and caregivers.	
Ask caregivers what they expect of their adolescent.	
Demonstrate age-appropriate interactions with the adolescent.	
Outline for caregivers the current stage of growth and development and the milestones to expect next.	
Explore the caregiver's concerns, especially sexual development, recreational drug and alcohol use, fiscal responsibility, adolescent's independence, discipline, and preparation for college or work.	Parent may need help in addressing issues and maintaining expectations for the adolescent.

▼

NURSING DIAGNOSIS: HIGH RISK FOR KNOWLEDGE DEFICIT (ADOLESCENT) CONCERNING EXPECTED GROWTH AND DEVELOPMENT

Risk Factors
- Rapid physical and social development
- Adults reluctant to discuss sexual development
- Misinformation from peers

Patient Outcomes
Adolescent will verbalize the expected developmental milestones for self.

Nursing Interventions	Rationales
Explore adolescent's concerns. Assess for pregnancy, STDs, alcohol/drug use.	Adolescents often present to health care worker with a complaint unrelated to true concerns: pregnancy, birth control, drugs, disease.
Provide privacy during discussions.	
Ensure confidentiality.	
Provide information and support without being judgmental.	
Help the adolescent to reach decisions that reflect his/her own values, rather than the values of the nurse, parents, or peers.	
Refer for individual or family counseling if necessary.	

▼

DISCHARGE PLANNING/CONTINUITY OF CARE

- Arrange referrals as needed
  - dietitian
  - social work
  - family therapist
  - psychiatrist/psychologist
  - self-help groups

- Communicate with school system concerning learning deficits.
- Refer for additional medical evaluation
  - gynecology: precocious/delayed puberty
  - endocrinology: delayed growth
- Follow up as needed.

REFERENCES

Amer, K., Augsut, G. P., & Robnett, M. A. (1992). *The nursing perspective: Monitoring and evaluation of growth* (pp. 21–20). Califon, NJ: Gardiner-Caldwell Syner Med.

Holt, K. S. (1991). *Child development diagnosis and assessment.* London: Butterworth-Heinemann.

Rice, M. S., & Gaines, S. K. (1992). Measurement of child temperament: Implications for researchers, clinicians and caregivers. *CHC, 21*(3), 177–183.

▼

GROWTH CHARTS

GIRLS: BIRTH TO 36 MONTHS
PHYSICAL GROWTH
NCHS PERCENTILES*

NAME _____ RECORD # _____

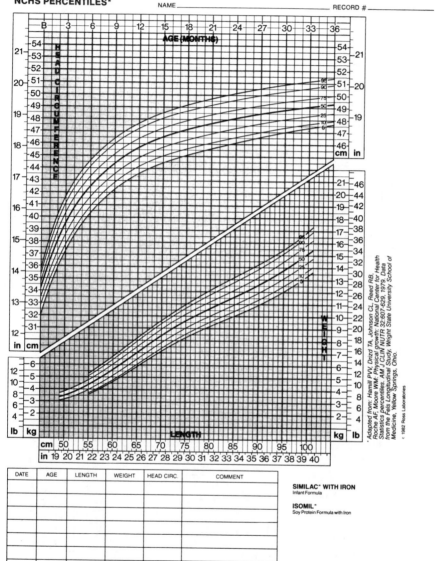

DATE	AGE	LENGTH	WEIGHT	HEAD CIRC.	COMMENT

Adapted from: Hamill PVV, Drizd TA, Johnson CL, Reed RB, Roche AF, Moore WM: Physical growth: National Center for Health Statistics percentiles. AM J CLIN NUTR 32:607-629, 1979. Data from the Fels Longitudinal Study, Wright State University School of Medicine, Yellow Springs, Ohio.

© 1982 Ross Laboratories

SIMILAC® WITH IRON
Infant Formula

ISOMIL®
Soy Protein Formula with Iron

Reprinted with permission
of Ross Laboratories

GIRLS: 2 TO 18 YEARS
PHYSICAL GROWTH
NCHS PERCENTILES*

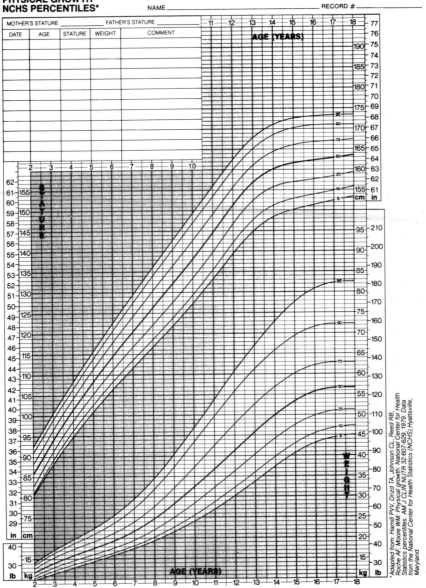

*Adapted from: Hamill PVV, Drizd TA, Johnson CL, Reed RB, Roche AF, Moore WM. Physical growth: National Center for Health Statistics percentiles. AM J CLIN NUTR 32:607-629, 1979. Data from the National Center for Health Statistics (NCHS), Hyattsville, Maryland.

© 1982 Ross Laboratories

**BOYS: BIRTH TO 36 MONTHS
PHYSICAL GROWTH
NCHS PERCENTILES***

NAME _____ _____ RECORD # _____

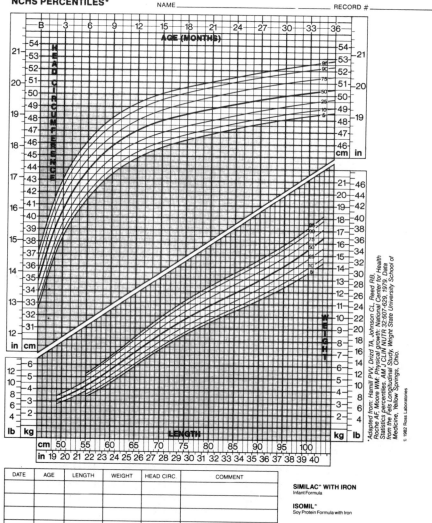

DATE	AGE	LENGTH	WEIGHT	HEAD CIRC.	COMMENT

*Adapted from: Hamill PVV, Drizd TA, Johnson CL, Reed RB, Roche AF, Moore WM: Physical growth: National Center for Health Statistics percentiles. AM J CLIN NUTR 32:607-629, 1979. Data from the Fels Longitudinal Study, Wright State University School of Medicine, Yellow Springs, Ohio.

© 1982 Ross Laboratories

SIMILAC* WITH IRON
Infant Formula

ISOMIL*
Soy Protein Formula with Iron

Reprinted with permission
of Ross Laboratories

BOYS: 2 TO 18 YEARS
PHYSICAL GROWTH
NCHS PERCENTILES*

NAME _____ RECORD # _____

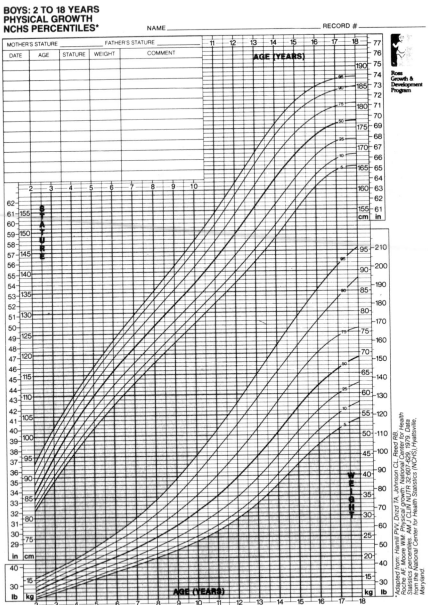

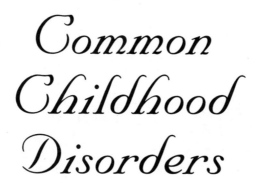

Common
Childhood
Disorders

▼

ABDOMINAL PAIN, ACUTE

Nedra Skale, RN, MS, CNA

Acute abdominal pain refers to the sudden onset of abdominal pain that may be severe or become progressively more severe.

ETIOLOGIES

- Appendicitis
- Meckel's diverticulum
- Ovarian cyst/torsion
- Constipation
- Pelvic inflammatory disease
- Sickle cell crisis
- Lead poisoning
- Enteritis
- Pancreatitis
- Henoch-Schönlein purpura
- Upper respiratory infection

CLINICAL MANIFESTATIONS

- Umbilical/periumbilical pain
- Back pain
- Colicky pain
- Rebound tenderness
- Abdominal distention
- Diarrhea
- Vomiting
- Fever
- Abdominal/rectal mass
- Headache

CLINICAL/DIAGNOSTIC FINDINGS

- Increased white blood cell count
- Heme-positive stool
- Positive stool culture
- Positive vaginal culture
- Increased serum lead level
- Positive abdominal films

▼

NURSING DIAGNOSIS: PAIN

Related To
- Infection
- Obstruction
- Inflammation

Defining Characteristics

The child reports a painful experience
Facial mask of pain
Crying, moaning
Guarded position
Increased pulse, blood pressure and respirations
Dilated pupils
Child does not want to be left alone
Restlessness

Patient Outcomes

The child will
- be diagnosed and treated.
- relate improvement in the pain.
- increase daily activities.

Nursing Interventions	Rationales
Ask the child to point to the area that hurts. Locate the site of maximal pain and radiation of the pain.	To more clearly define origin of pain.
Determine the intensity of the pain by asking the child to rate the pain using an age-appropriate scale.	The child's description will help with differential diagnosis.

Nursing Interventions

Determine the severity of illness:
1. Mildly ill children have pain but it does not interfere with normal activities.

Rationales

Henoch-Schönlein purpura—This is a diffuse vasculitis that begins with colicky pain. There can be right lower quadrant tenderness.
Upper respiratory infections—Infections with pulmonary infiltrates often are associated with abdominal pain. The fever is higher, however, than that found in appendicitis. The child also may have enlarged lymph nodes, headache, and muscle pain.
Lead poisoning—Attacks of abdominal pain usually are colicky, with constipation and vomiting. On physical examination the child will be irritable, with intermittent pain. There are no localized findings.

Nursing Interventions

2. Moderately ill children have pain that interferes with normal activity or have signs of infection or systemic illness.

Rationales

Appendicitis—This is the most common acute surgical emergency in childhood. It occurs in all age groups but is most common during later childhood and early adulthood. The mean age range in the pediatric population is 6–10 years, but appendicitis does occur in newborns and infants. Pain is progressive; it begins as periumbilical and radiates to the right lower quadrant. Rebound and McBurney's point tenderness usually is seen.

Torsion of an ovary, ovarian cyst, or teratoma—These usually cause lower abdominal pain and tenderness, but the onset of pain is sudden and often a mass can be felt on rectal examination.

Constipation—This may cause cecal distention and pain in the right side of the abdomen.

Pelvic inflammatory disease—This usually begins with lower abdominal pain, high fever, and a purulent vaginal discharge following a menstrual period.

Enteric infections—Infections such as shigellosis and salmonella can cause severe abdominal pain, fever, and diarrhea that is profuse and watery.

Pancreatitis—This will cause sudden onset of upper abdominal pain with vomiting and distention. The pain often radiates to the back. Children are most comfortable sitting in bed, leaning forward.

Nursing Interventions	Rationales
3. Severely ill children have signs of peritonitis or intestinal obstruction and may have altered mental status.	*Sickle cell anemia*—These children have abdominal crises with severe pain. They appear chronically ill with anemia. The pain is more severe than that of appendicitis, with abdominal distention and tenderness. The abdominal pain usually subsides within 8–12 hours with adequate treatment. *Meckel's diverticulum (perforated)*—The diverticulum is the most common congenital anomaly of the intestine. It is present in 2% of the population. It is usually within 2 feet of the ileocecal valve and is usually not more than 2 inches in length. Bloody stools and umbilical pain usually are more severe in children under the age of 2 years, and boys are affected more often than girls. It is also seen more often in Caucasians than blacks. Appendicitis and enteritis can become increasingly severe.
Determine the child's concept of the cause of the pain. Ask the child what makes the pain better and what makes it worse.	

Nursing Interventions	**Rationales**
Note signs of peritoneal irritation, such as ileopsoas rigidity, pain with external thigh rotation, pain with jarring movements, difficulty walking, or referred pain to the neck or shoulder.	If epigastric pain exists, consider • peptic ulcer • hiatal hernia • gastroesophageal reflux • esophagitis • pancreatitis If right upper quadrant pain exists, consider • constipation • hepatitis • liver abscess or tumor • cholecystitis • cholangitis If mild, diffuse periumbilical or left-sided pain exists, consider • constipation • food poisoning • pharyngitis/upper respiratory infection • muscle strain • gastroenteritis If right lower quadrant pain exists, consider • appendicitis • Henoch-Schönlein purpura If intermittent, crampy pain exists, consider • intussusception • lead poisoning
Note associated symptoms of urinary tract involvement (dysuria, frequency) and the presence of fever, vomiting, diarrhea, rectal bleeding, jaundice, or weight loss.	
Identify precipitating factors, including constipation, trauma, medications, sickle cell disease, menses, pregnancy, or past abdominal surgery.	
Explore the possibility of dietary intolerance contributing to the abdominal pain.	

Nursing Interventions	**Rationales**
Identify food that the child feels causes him/her problems.	Suspect lactose intolerance when symptoms of cramping, bloating, flatus, or diarrhea develop about 2 hours after the ingestion of milk or milk products. A lactose-free diet for 4 weeks may be helpful in determining intolerance.
Once a definitive diagnosis is made: 1. Inform the family of the diagnosis and the cause. If surgery is indicated, reinforce the need for the surgery and what to anticipate prior to the surgery. Teach the family about the expected postoperative recovery.	
2. If surgery is not indicated, assess the educational needs of the child and family as they relate to the reason for the pain and the treatment suggested.	
3. Explain the pain source to the child using verbal and sensory explanations. Reinforce to the child that he/she is not being punished.	Magical thinking in a young child may lead him/her to believe he/she is being punished for thoughts/wishes.
4. Provide pain-relieving measures specific to diagnosis.	

▼

DISCHARGE PLANNING/CONTINUITY OF CARE

- Refer to
  - pediatric surgeon
  - dietitian
- Follow up in office when needed.
- Explain signs and symptoms necessitating emergent care.

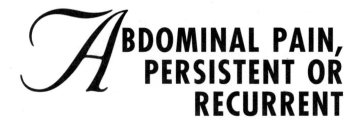BDOMINAL PAIN, PERSISTENT OR RECURRENT

Nedra Skale, RN, MS, CNA

Persistent or recurrent abdominal pain can be defined as acute episodes of pain occurring at least monthly for a minimum of 3 months in a row. It is most common in children ages 10–12 years. One in 10 children comes to the doctor because of recurrent abdominal pain.

Organic

This cause is most likely if the pain is present consistently in the same place and can be well localized by the child. The pain usually awakens the child at night and is not related to a stressful situation.

Psychogenic

This cause is most likely if the child is female and between the ages of 9 and 14. The pain described is vague or diffuse and ill-defined in both nature and location. The child is not ill. The pain does not awaken the child at night. Other symptoms often associated with this type of abdominal pain are pallor, dizziness, and headache.

ETIOLOGIES

- Infection
- Organic disease
- Obstruction
- Ulcer
- Stress
- Situational crises

CLINICAL MANIFESTATIONS

Organic
- Point tenderness
- Rebound tenderness
- Abdominal rigidity

- Fever
- Rash
- Diarrhea
- Vomiting
- Peritoneal signs

Psychogenic
- Diffuse pain
- Vague location
- Vague complaints
- Sleeps without pain
- Dizziness
- Headache
- Pallor
- No other signs of illness

CLINICAL/DIAGNOSTIC FINDINGS: ORGANIC

- Weight loss
- Heme-positive stools
- Hematuria
- Positive abdominal films/ultrasound
- Positive endoscopic exam

▼

NURSING DIAGNOSIS: PAIN

Related To (see Clinical Manifestations)

Defining Characteristics
The child reports a painful experience
Facial mask of pain
Guarded position
Increased pulse, blood pressure and respirations
Dilated pupils
Child does not want to be left alone
Restlessness

Patient Outcomes
The child will
- relate improvement in the pain and an increase in daily activities.
- identify activities that increase or decrease the pain.

Nursing Interventions	Rationales
Identify predisposing conditions such as menses, sickle cell disease, or food allergies. Provide treatment for underlying conditions.	
If no underlying condition exists, assess the child's degree of illness and pain. 1. Determine the child's concept of the cause of the pain. 2. Ask the child what makes the pain better and what makes it worse. 3. Determine the intensity of the pain by asking the child to rate the pain using an age-appropriate scale. 4. Ask the child to point to the area that hurts. 5. Document the presence of point tenderness, rebound tenderness or abdominal rigidity.	Children with mild illness have pain that interferes with normal activity but is not incapacitating. Children with moderate illness have signs of infection or other systematic disorders. Children with severe illness have peritoneal signs: pain that prevents walking, intestinal obstruction, prior abdominal surgery, or necrotizing enterocolitis.
Assess for signs of organic disease: history of bloody stools, weight loss, perianal lesions, fever, rash, pain radiating to the back or shoulder, abnormal laboratory results, nocturnal pain, or a positive family history of ulcer disease.	*Epigastric pain* suggests peptic ulcer disease, hiatal hernia, gastroesophageal reflux, esophagitis, or pancreatis. *Right upper quadrant* pain suggests hepatitis, liver abscess or tumor, Fitz-Hugh–Curtis syndrome, cholecystitis, cholangitis or choledochal cyst.
Determine associated gastrointestinal manifestations.	
Determine extraintestinal manifestations such as fever, rash, weight loss, hematuria, limb pains, headaches, nausea, pallor, vomiting, and perspiration.	Associated manifestations assist with differentiating organic disease and diminish the likelihood of psychogenic disorder.
Explain tests that will be needed to determine organic cause: 1. x-ray 2. ultrasound 3. endoscopy	

Nursing Interventions	Rationales
Explain that pain medications must be withheld until differential diagnosis is confirmed.	Pain medications can mask developing symptoms of organic disease.
Provide nonpharmacological pain control measures: 1. toys 2. hold/rock 3. encourage parent presence	
Assure parent and child that, once diagnosis is confirmed, pain medication will be prescribed.	

▼

NURSING DIAGNOSIS: ALTERED FAMILY PROCESSES

Related To
- Child's illness
- Chronic disease
- Change in family structure
- Psychological disorder

Defining Characteristics
Change in the child's ability to function
Parents unable to meet the physical and/or emotional needs of the child
Family unable to adapt constructively to crisis

Patient Outcomes
- The family can recognize the problems of the individual members in terms meaningful to the whole family.
- The family can demonstrate constructive communication and interaction.
- The child and/or family will express knowledge of the problem and the solutions proposed by the medical staff.

Nursing Interventions	Rationales
Determine the functional level of impairment, the anxiety level of the child and family, the family history of functional illness, and the presence of stress in the child's life.	The family's lack of concern about the impact of recurrent abdominal pain on the child's life suggests a psychogenic disorder. The child usually has low self-esteem and very few friends. There may be an inability to cope with change or stressful situations. Academic performance is low.
Note any crisis, such as a recent divorce, illness, or death in the family or of a friend; a move; or a fight with a friend or parents.	
Counsel the child and family in stress reduction techniques. Counsel the family on how to minimize secondary gain in relation to abdominal pain.	
Assess the educational needs of the child and family as related to the reason for the pain and the treatment suggested.	
Explain the pain source to the child using verbal and sensory explanations. Reinforce to the child that he/she is not being punished.	Magical thinking in a young child may lead him/her to believe he/she is being punished for thoughts/wishes.
Explain to the parents the need for honest explanations to promote trust.	

▼

DISCHARGE PLANNING/CONTINUITY OF CARE

- Refer to mental health professional if problem is psychogenic.
- Refer to dietitian for assistance in food selection/preparation and determining allergies to certain foods.
- Refer to pediatric surgeon for treatment of organic dysfunction.

$\mathcal{A}$CNE

Nedra Skale, RN, MS, CNA

Acne vulgaris occurs when hormonal changes of puberty stimulate the sebaceous gland to produce excessive sebum. The sebaceous ducts become obstructed when sebum mixes with the epithelial cells to form keratin. Keratin impactions are called comedomes. The hair follicle becomes colonized with bacteria that initiate an inflammatory response that ruptures the canal wall and produces a papulopustule. Inflammatory acne presents with raised red papules, pustules, or cystic lesions. Cystic acne develops when pustules rupture under the skin and become lined with epithelium. This process produces scarring that is permanent.

ETIOLOGIES

- Increased androgen levels
- Infection

CLINICAL MANIFESTATIONS

- Raised, red papules
- Pustules
- Cysts
- Blackheads

CLINICAL/DIAGNOSTIC FINDINGS

Laboratory tests are not usually performed.

▼

NURSING DIAGNOSIS: IMPAIRED SKIN INTEGRITY

Related To
- Inflammatory process
- Obstructed sebaceous ducts

Defining Characteristics

Denuded skin

Excretions and secretions

Lesions

- noninflamed—open comedones (blackheads) with openings that are discolored, or closed comedones (whiteheads) with no visible opening
- inflamed—papules, pustules, nodules, and cysts

Erythema

Drainage

Patient Outcomes

- Infection will be controlled.
- Scar formation will be prevented.
- Excessive sebaceous gland activity will be controlled.

Nursing Interventions	Rationales
Instruct the child and family on the correct administration of the treatment prescribed.	
Benzoyl peroxide 1. Apply a thin layer once or twice a day over the entire face, avoiding the eyes and mouth. 2. Leave this layer on all day. 3. Use water-based moisturizers to help with dryness and irritation. 4. Use in 4–6 week trials.	This gel, liquid, or cream has an antibacterial action, reduces fatty acid concentrations, and has co-medolytic activity.
Topical antibiotic 1. Apply a thin layer as directed by the physician (usually 2–3 times a day).	Erythromycin, tetracycline, clindamycin, or meclocycline may be used if the benzoyl peroxide treatment fails. Antibiotics kill bacteria harbored on skin.

Nursing Interventions	Rationales

Retin A (tretinoin)
1. Apply to the face at night, avoiding the eyes, nose, and mouth.
2. Instruct the child to avoid sun exposure by using a sunscreen with a protective factor of at least 15.
3. Anticipate that the acne may worsen initially.
4. Use for at least a 6–12-week course (may be necessary before a response is apparent).

This acts by preventing comedome formation, opening closed comedomes, and increasing blood flow to the skin. Retin A is drying and irritating to the skin.

Oral antibiotics
1. Take erythromycin or tetracycline 500 mg orally twice a day as the usual starting dose.
2. If there is improvement, decrease the dose and frequency.
3. Take erythromycin with food.
4. Take tetracycline on an empty stomach to aid in its absorption.

These are used to treat inflammatory acne that has failed to respond to topical treatments.

Accutane (isotretinoin)

This is used in cystic acne that is unresponsive to the above treatments.

1. Explain that Accutane should not be used in pregnant or nursing mothers or in sexually active teens who are not on an acceptable birth control method.
2. Take 0.5–2.0 mg/kg orally, usually in two divided doses daily for 15–20 weeks.
3. Inform of possible side effects: dry skin, epistaxis, arthralgias, hepatitis, depression, elevation in serum triglycerides, and fatigue.

Accutane can cause severe birth defects.

▼

NURSING DIAGNOSIS: BODY IMAGE DISTURBANCE

Related To skin lesions

Defining Characteristics
Negative feelings about body/face
Withdrawl from social contacts
Not looking at face
Staring at face excessively

Patient Outcomes
The child will
- verbalize positive statements of body image.
- maintain an appropriate level of social involvement.

Nursing Interventions	Rationales
Assess the child's concerns about facial blemishes.	To the teen, any noticable lesion can single them out from their peers. They can have concerns about acne and sexual relations, venereal diseases, and the concept of being unclean. Reassurance can relieve these fears.
Emphasize that the teen years are an important physical and emotional life transition. Acknowledge the normalcy of these concerns.	The acne lesions need not be an excuse to avoid friends or activities. Explore job opportunities and other after-school interests with the teen.
Assist child to recognize positive aspects about self and the body (i.e., physically fit, good sense of humor, hard worker).	
Assess the child's normal habits as they relate to cleansing of the skin.	
Educate the child about proper washing with mild soap and avoiding excessive scrubbing.	Too vigorous scrubbing damages the skin and may be a focus of infection.

Nursing Interventions	**Rationales**
Educate the child that the use of cosmetics and oil-based lubricants should be limited or avoided and that cosmetics should not be left on the face overnight.	It is important that the child and family receive an explanation of the condition because acne commonly is associated with myths and treatment influenced by commercial advertising. The family must know the rationale underlying the treatment and the lengthy course of the disease so they will not have unrealistic expectations concerning the progress of therapy.

▼

DISCHARGE PLANNING/CONTINUITY OF CARE

- Refer to dermatologist.
- Follow up as needed.

ANEMIA

Susan Geoghegan, RN, BSN

Anemia is the reduction of red cell mass: the decrease in number of circulating red blood cells (RBCs) and decreased hemoglobin concentration. Normal hemoglobin levels are age dependent, highest at birth (16.5 g/dL) and lowest to age 3 months (normal nadir).

Although anemia can be transient and benign, persistent symptoms require careful evaluation. Any child presenting with obvious bleeding should be assessed and treated for shock, then referred for hospitalization.

ETIOLOGIES

- Bleeding (gastrointestinal, hematuria)
- Decreased red cell production (aplastic or hypoplastic anemias)
- Increased destruction of red cells (hemolytic anemias)
- Iron deficiency
- Prematurity

CLINICAL MANIFESTATIONS

- Abnormal growth and development
- Pallor, jaundice, headache
- Fever, weight loss, fatigue
- Petechiae, purpura
- Tachypnea, tachycardia
- Diaphoresis, hypotension
- Hepatosplenomegaly
- Lymphadenopathy
- Obvious bleeding

CLINICAL/DIAGNOSTIC FINDINGS

- Abnormal red cell count
  - newborn: < 3.6 million/mm^3
  - 1 month: < 3.0 million/mm^3

- 1 year: < 4.0 million/mm^3
- childhood: < 4.0 million/mm^3
- adolescence: < 4.0 million/mm^3 (female)
- adolescence: < 4.5 million/mm^3 (male)
- Abnormal hemoglobin
  - newborn: < 14 g/dL
  - 1 month: < 10 g/dL
  - 1 year: < 11 g/dL
  - childhood: < 13 g/dL
  - adolescence: < 12 g/dL (female)
  - adolescence: < 12.5 g/dL (male)
- Decreased serum ferritin/iron
- Heme-positive urine/stool

▼

NURSING DIAGNOSIS: ACTIVITY INTOLERANCE

Related To
- Anemia
- Poor tissue perfusion

Defining Characteristics

Verbalized fatigue
Weakness
Sleepiness
Tachycardia or dyspnea on exertion
Child unable to keep up with peers

Patient Outcomes

- Child will be wakeful and tolerate normal activities for age without fatigue.
- Child's vital signs will be within normal range for age after exertion.

Nursing Interventions	Rationales
Assess for clinical manifestations/ defining characteristics.	
Assess family history/origins.	Disorder may be inherited.
Assess diet for iron consumption, especially in infants and toddlers.	
Assess laboratory values: 1. hemoglobin/hematocrit 2. RBC/white blood cell count with differential.	To assist in determining differential diagnosis.

Nursing Interventions	Rationales
Assess hydration.	Increased blood volume with normal RBC mass does not indicate anemia. Dehydration can mask reduced RBC mass.
Explain further testing required for differential diagnosis: blood smear, reticulocyte count, Coombs' test, haptoglobin, bilirubin levels, bone marrow aspiration.	Medical treatment depends on type of anemia/etiology.
Discuss home care measures that can be implemented without specific diagnosis:	
1. Encourage frequent rest periods.	Rest is necessary to decrease demand on circulating RBCs.
2. Limit play/sport activities to those that do not tax respiratory/cardiac response.	
3. Provide balanced meals, with increase in iron (Fe)-containing foods and/or provide iron supplement.	Infants and toddlers require about 8 mg. of iron/day because of rapid growth and blood volume expansion (see Nutrition, p 285).
4. Maintain a safe environment.	This is necessary to prevent accidental bruising/bleeding.
Refer immediately if cardiac decompensation is suspected.	Decreasing cardiac output is life threatening.

▼

NURSING DIAGNOSIS: HIGH RISK FOR INFECTION

Risk Factors
- Poor skin condition
- Anemia with poor perfusion
- Decreased immune response

Patient Outcomes
Child will not develop infection, as evidenced by afebrile state, no wounds or drainage.

Nursing Interventions	Rationales
Assess for signs of infection: 1. fever (hypothermia in very young infants) 2. pain 3. swelling, redness 4. open wounds 5. drainage	
Instruct parents to minimize risks by 1. providing good skin and oral hygiene. 2. maintaining balanced diet. 3. practicing good hand washing. 4. avoiding exposure to high-risk situations (i.e., crowds, school, day care). If there is significant risk, alternative schooling may need to be arranged.	Bacterial and viral infections are transmitted easily in the close contact of classrooms.
Teach parents signs of infection and how to measure child's temperature.	
Instruct parents to give child antibiotics if ordered. (See Idiopathic Thrombocytopenic Purpura, p 187; Hemophilia, p 167; and Sickle Cell Anemia, p 242)	

▼

DISCHARGE PLANNING/CONTINUITY OF CARE

- Follow-up determined by differential diagnosis/treatment/severity of anemia.
- Facilitate consults:
  – hematologist
  – immunologist

ASTHMA

Michele Knoll Puzas, RNC, MHPE

Bronchial asthma, also called reactive airway disease, is the obstruction of the tracheobronchial tree as a result of mucosal edema and bronchial spasms.

ETIOLOGIES

- Allergic response
- Infection
- Emotional response

CLINICAL MANIFESTATIONS

- Expiratory wheezing
- Inspiratory and expiratory wheezing in infant
- Rales, hyperresonance
- Retractions, including intercostal and suprasternal in infants
- Nasal flaring
- Use of accessory muscles

CLINICAL/DIAGNOSTIC FINDINGS

- Eosinophilia
- Eosinophils in sputum
- Decreased peak expiratory flow rate
- Hyperinflation seen on chest film

▼

NURSING DIAGNOSIS: INEFFECTIVE AIRWAY CLEARANCE

Related To
- Bronchial edema
- Bronchospasms

Defining Characteristics
Dyspnea
Wheezing
Nonproductive cough
Tachycardia
Restlessness

Patient Outcome
The child will breathe without difficulty.

Nursing Interventions	Rationales
Assess for past history of wheezing episodes, including: 1. recent upper respiratory infection 2. recent exposure to allergens 3. exercise-related episodes	
Assess lung sounds.	
Observe for retractions, nasal flaring, cough and use of accessory muscles.	
Ask the child to describe how he/she feels.	The older child will be able to describe a tightness in his/her chest.
Assess heart rate/rhythm.	
Assess hydration.	Children dehydrate quickly as a result of the insensible water loss of rapid respiration.
Obtain pulse oximetry reading if available.	
Administer humidified oxygen.	Necessary to prevent or reverse hypoxemia and reduce water loss.

Nursing Interventions	Rationales
Encourage oral fluids, if able, or begin intravenous (IV) hydration.	Rehydration is necessary to thin mucus secretions and ease respiration.

Administer medications.
1. Bronchodilators
  • epinephrine hydrochloride, 1:1000, SC, 0.01/mg/kg (do not exceed 0.3 mg). Repeat twice. Monitor for tachycardia, tremors, anxiety.
  • theophylline, PO, loading dose, 6 mg/kg. Maintain serum theophylline level at 10–20 mcg/mL. Monitor for stomach upset, nausea, vomiting, headache, restlessness, insomnia.
  • albuterol, inhaler, 1 inhalation < 12 years old, 2 inhalations > 12 years old, every 4–6 hr. Monitor for palpitations, tachycardia, nausea, headache, dizziness, dry throat.
Bronchodilators should be continued for a few days after symptoms subside to decrease chance of recurrence.
2. Corticosteroids, inhaled and/or orally (IV only in acute attacks): 1 inhalation 15 min *after* albuterol.
	Inhaled corticosteroids cause less adrenal hypofunction but, like oral or IV routes, inhaled corticosteroid doses should be tapered over 5–7 days and not abruptly discontinued.

Refer for hospitalization if improvement is not seen.	
Explain all medications to be taken at home.	Depending on the severity of the child's illness and his/her response to treatment, home medications may range from a few days of continued bronchodilator with or without steriod to long-term bronchodilation therapy. Long-term steroid use is avoided because of adverse effects.

Nursing Interventions	Rationales
Teach child how to use inhaler, caution against overuse and adverse effects.	Inhalers should be cleaned daily to prevent fungal infections of the mouth, pharynx, and larynx.
Teach parent how to use a nebulizer with infant/toddler.	
Provide information about control of environmental allergens specific to the child's needs.	Controlling the child's environment may be helpful in limiting the number and severity of attacks.

▼

DISCHARGE PLANNING/CONTINUITY OF CARE

- Explain signs and symptoms requiring immediate follow-up: persistent wheezing, chest pain, cyanosis, fever, increasing dyspnea.
- Have child return for serum theophylline level 2–3 days after beginning medication.
- Encourage the use of Medic-Alert or other identification indicating diagnosis and medications.
- Provide information about support groups, asthma camp, American Lung Association.
- Refer for respiratory therapy, allergy testing, dietary consult.

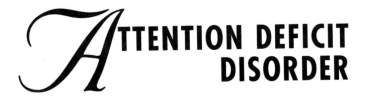

ATTENTION DEFICIT DISORDER

Kathleen Scharer, RN, MS, CS, FAAN

Attention deficit disorder (ADD) affects the child's ability to modulate attention for his/her mental age. It usually is accompanied by impulsivity.

ETIOLOGY

Based on current research, the sleep center of the brain is somewhat damaged, causing the child to be constantly on the verge of sleep. The behaviors of the child are designed to prevent him/her from fully sleeping.

CLINICAL MANIFESTATIONS

- Inability to attend to tasks or activities. EXAMPLES:
  - often fails to complete something he/she starts
  - easily distracted from activity, including play activities
  - often appears not to listen
  - cannot concentrate on the task at hand for more than short periods
- Demonstrates impulsivity. EXAMPLES:
  - frequently acts before thinking
  - has difficulty waiting for a turn
  - frequently alternates among activities, without completing any
  - inability to organize tasks
  - requires frequent to constant monitoring by adults
- Hyperactivity that may serve to maintain wakefulness may or may not be present. EXAMPLES:
  - moves about excessively
  - cannot sit still for very long
  - when required to stay in a chair, fidgets constantly
  - behavior seems driven
- Disorder usually is apparent before age 3.
- Specific learning disabilities may or may not be present.

CLINICAL/DIAGNOSTIC FINDINGS

May have abnormal electroencephalogram

▼

NURSING DIAGNOSIS: IMPAIRED SOCIAL INTERACTION

Related To inability to attend to subject for extended time

Defining Characteristics

Verbalized or observed inability to receive or communicate a sense of belonging, caring, or interest
Observed use of unsuccessful social interaction behaviors
Dysfunctional interactions with peers, family, or others
Inability to organize and remain focused until a task is completed
Easily distracted from interactions because of short attention span
Often appears not to be listening or not to hear what is said to him/her
Disruptive classroom behavior because of attentional difficulties
Play often is disrupted by limited attention span or impulsivity

Patient Outcome

The child demonstrates improved ability to interact and play with others socially, as evidenced by forming and satisfactorily maintaining one relationship with a peer.

Nursing Interventions	Rationales
Asess child's limitations and strengths in interactions with peers and adults. Determine if skill deficits exist or if inability to attend is primary cause of impaired social interactions.	
Assess parental responses to child's behavior with others.	Parents inadvertently may be reinforcing less desirable behaviors and diminishing child's self-esteem.
Assess typical duration of attention in interactions.	
Decrease environmental stimulation that may distract child during social interactions.	

Nursing Interventions	Rationales
Provide positive reinforcement for appropriate interaction. Refocus child if distracted.	Child needs encouragement for appropriate responses to learn social skills.
Teach child specific, age-appropriate social skills where deficits exist and provide practice opportunities.	
Educate parents about child's disorder and need for assistance in developing relationships.	
Teach parents methods to refocus distracted child in positive manner. For example, when child leaves playmate in the middle of a game and wants to begin a new activity, parents can gently point out to the child that his/her peer is wishing to finish the game and he/she needs to complete the game before beginning something new.	
Refer child and family to psychotherapist for therapy and possibly for medication.	Stimulant medication may be required to increase the child's ability to attend to schoolwork.
Educate the parents about the child's need for a thorough educational assessment and the possibility of obtaining special educational assistance even prior to kindergarten.	Early educational intervention can help the child compensate for any learning disabilities.

▼

NURSING DIAGNOSIS: SLEEP PATTERN DISTURBANCE

Related To neurological disturbance

Defining Characteristics
Awakening earlier than parents desire
Verbal complaints (by parents) of difficulty in falling sleep
Interrupted sleep

Patient Outcomes
The child will
• go to bed at a set time and fall asleep within 30 min.

- remain in bed each morning until a specified time.
- obtain 8–10 hr of uninterrupted sleep per night.

Nursing Interventions	Rationales
Assess child's usual sleep patterns. Have parent keep a diary for 1 month that includes 1. start of bedtime rituals. 2. nature (bath, snack, story, etc.) and duration of rituals until child is in bed. 3. number of times child is out of bed before falling asleep. 4. number of awakenings during night. 5. length of time to resume sleeping and time of awakening.	Knowledge of type and degree of problems is necessary for planning care and measuring improvement.
Reassess problem using the diary technique periodically to assess improvements and evaluate interventions.	
Teach parents about the nature of the child's disorder, including sleep disturbances.	When a child is difficult to get to sleep and sleeps an insufficient amount of time, parents often suffer from sleep disruption as a result. This may interfere with their ability to manage the child or they may begin to feel the behavior is intentional.
Assist the parents to develop and follow a consistent bedtime schedule, reasonable rituals, and wake up time for the child. Rituals may include a hot bath, backrub, story, and soft relaxing music through headphones. Once in bed, the child should not be allowed out of bed.	Child will learn to fall asleep easier if there are no deviations in the bedtime routine.
Prohibit snacks or beverages with caffeine from dinner time to bedtime. An even earlier limit may be required for younger children with earlier bedtimes.	Caffeine promotes wakefullness. It can be found in many children's snack foods.

Nursing Interventions	Rationales
Assist the parents in developing a plan for sleep interruptions and for early morning wakening: 1. Utilize the same music tape used at bedtime. 2. The morning plan might include that the child can play quietly in bed but cannot get out of bed.	

▼

NURSING DIAGNOSIS: CHRONIC LOW SELF-ESTEEM

Related To
• Repeated negative feedback about behavior
• Skill deficits in interaction processes
• Inadequate repertoire of compensating mechanisms

Defining Characteristics
Self-negating verbalizations
Evaluates self as unable to deal with events
Expressions of shame and guilt
Frequent lack of success in school or other life events
Rationalizes away/rejects positive feedback and exaggerates negative feedback about self
Is aware of inability to organize and remain focused until a task is completed
Experiences self as different from other children; as damaged in some way

Patient Outcomes
• The child will verbalize positive feeling about himself/herself.
• The parents will demonstrate knowledge of the child's disorder in setting appropriate limits and structuring the environment to facilitate the child's developing increased control over his/her behavior.

Nursing Interventions	Rationales
Identify factors that contribute to the child's low self-esteem.	
Identify child's perception of any strengths or special qualities the child values.	These may be used to build on in designing the plan of care.

Nursing Interventions	Rationales
Assess parents' style of limit setting and their structuring of the child's environment.	Parents may need information about ways to better manage their child.
Assess changes in child's feelings about himself/herself over time.	This will serve as a measure of the improvement in the child's self-esteem.
Assess if any other individuals may be contributing to the child's diminished self esteem, such as a teacher.	If the child frequently is being demeaned by someone, work needs to be done with that individual.
Assist the child in developing more effective social skills.	Poor social skills contribute to the child's diminished self-esteem.
Educate the parents about the use of positive reinforcement and ignoring less desirable behavior.	
Teach the parents to structure the child's environment and required tasks to provide the likelihood of success.	If tasks and the environment are simplified and less distracting, the child's successes will enhance self-esteem.
Encourage the parents to foster those activities in which the child has most successes.	Increased successes enhance self-esteem.
Utilize play and art expression for mastery of difficult experiences.	A sense of mastery of difficult situation increases the child's self-esteem.
Work with the parents to develop a plan for dealing with others about the special needs of their child.	Parents must serve as an advocate for their child.

▼

DISCHARGE PLANNING/CONTINUITY OF CARE

- Refer to psychotherapist for therapy and possible medication.
- Refer to educational specialist for assessment of and intervention for any specific learning disabilities.
- Encourage parents to explore special activities for children with ADD, such as special camps or park activities. These provide opportunities for the child to participate and succeed in activities with adults who understand their difficulties.

$\mathscr{B}$RONCHOPULMONARY DYSPLASIA

Diana Stephens, RNC, NP

Bronchopulmonary dysplasia (BPD) is a disease process, common among preterm infants, resulting in chronic changes in lung parenchyma that include scarring, atelectasis, and air trapping. This care plan will focus on the care needs of infants who have been discharged home on oxygen/ventilator therapy and are being evaluated in a follow-up clinic.

ETIOLOGIES

- Prematurity
- Barotrauma
- Oxygen toxicity
- Inadequate nutrition

CLINICAL MANIFESTATIONS

- Cyanosis or pallor
- Altered breath sounds
- Tachycardia
- Tachypnea
- Pulse oximetry $\leq 90\%$
- Abnormal chest films

▼

NURSING DIAGNOSIS: INEFFECTIVE BREATHING

Related To
- Disease process
- Fatigue
- Pulmonary edema
- Infection

- Discomfort
- Bronchospasm

Defining Characteristics
Beyond baseline tachypnea, retractions, nasal flaring
Wheezing, inspiratory crackles, coarse rales
Impaired ability to feed orally
Persistent hypoxia (oxygen saturation by pulse oximeter < 88%)
Difficulty in consoling from an agitated state
More easily fatigued
Edema
Cyanosis

Patient Outcomes
Infant will maintain optimal respiratory status as evidenced by:
- breathing rate/depth within expected limits
- oxygen saturation above 92%
- no evidence of retractions, nasal flaring

Nursing Interventions	Rationales
Obtain thorough history of infant's status at home since last visit or phone conversation regarding respiratory patterns, tolerance to activity, sleep patterns, and feeding abilities.	Having well-documented baseline examinations of patient and responses to activity and therapies is necessary to ensure that ongoing assessments are accurate and changes in exam are readily diagnosed
Evaluate oxygen need based on this history and observation of infant status during visit: 1. Assess oxygen saturation with pulse oximeter at rest, during feeding, and during activity. 2. Assess respiratory status over a period of time. 3. Assess pulses and perfusion.	
Increase oxygen delivery, when necessary, to achieve oxygen saturations of > 92%. Obtain blood gas if condition does not improve after increasing fraction of inspired oxygen.	Oxygen saturations nearing 90% or under are indicative of impending hypoxia and hypoxic events.
Observe infant's behaviors and responses to care interventions.	

Nursing Interventions	Rationales
Review prescribed pharmacological therapy, dosing, and schedules.	These patients may be on a variety of drug regimens designed to improve their respiratory status: diuretics, oral and inhaled preparations of steroids, and oral and inhaled preparations of bronchodilators. It is imperative that the beneficial effects of therapies be evaluated so that dosing regimens are optimized for each patient.
Observe caretakers' responses to infant's changes in oxygenation and their ease with intervening as appropriate.	
Consider urine hematest as part of evaluation for urinary tract infection or hypercalciuria.	Hypercalciuria is a known side effect for BPD patients on chronic furosemide therapy. It is associated with renal stone formation and urinary tract infections and can be a source of discomfort that might compromise respiratory status.

▼

NURSING DIAGNOSIS: ALTERED NUTRITION—LESS THAN BODY REQUIREMENTS

Related To
- Fatigue associated with nipple feedings
- Increased energy expenditures resulting from increased work of breathing
- Limited capabilities for increasing caloric intake
- Gastroesophageal reflux (recurrent episodes of emesis/irritability)

Defining Characteristics
Failure to gain weight
Chronic irritability

Patient Outcomes
- The infant will maintain optimal nutritional status, as evidenced by weight gain.
- The parents will verbalize understanding of the treatment plan.

Nursing Interventions	Rationales
Assess weight, length, and head circumference routinely on visits and maintain growth chart.	
Document feeding volumes, schedule, and route with each visit.	Most infants with BPD are difficult to feed. However, they can thrive, especially in the home environment.
Maintain caloric intake history. Assess for signs of gastroesophageal reflux.	
Establish feeding routine/regimen/route appropriate for this infant. Include dietitian and parents in development of nutritional plan. Assess tolerance to plan.	At home, the infant has a consistent caregiver familiar with the infant, who recognizes infant's feeding cues and can provide a relaxed, unhurried setting for feeding. These caregivers, when given the necessary support of a nutrition team, can develop the best feeding regimen for their infant.
Supplement nutrition with caloric additives to formula per physician and dietitian recommendations.	
Enlist occupational or speech therapist to work with the infant's feeding process if necessary.	A change in feeding technique may improve intake.
Perform periodic blood work for electrolyte analysis, nutritional assays.	

▼

NURSING DIAGNOSIS: HIGH RISK FOR INFECTION

Risk Factors
- Damaged airways or tenacious secretions that promote bacterial invasion
- Poor nutritional status
- Impaired immune response

Patient Outcomes

Parents will verbalize
- understanding of prevention strategies to reduce infant's risk of infection.
- signs/symptoms related to infection.

Nursing Interventions	Rationales
Assess health status of household, especially with regard to respiratory illnesses.	
Educate caregivers on infant's increased risk for infections and need for limiting exposure.	Because of the infant's damaged airway and thick secretions, infection occurs easily and could be life threatening.
Instruct caregivers in importance of hygiene, especially careful handwashing.	
Promote optimal nutrition and weight gain.	This will help the infant to combat infections.
Ensure administration of immunizations per normal schedule.	To minimize risk of devastating respiratory complications caused by illness.
Instruct parents in signs and symptoms of infection/respiratory compromise: 1. respiratory distress symptoms, wheezing 2. tachycardia 3. cough 4. lethargy 5. sustained irritability 6. persistent fever 7. cyanosis	

▼

NURSING DIAGNOSIS: IMPAIRED PHYSICAL MOBILITY

Related To
- Long-term hospitalization
- Extreme prematurity and very low birth weight
- Difficulties/impairments in infant handling

Defining Characteristics
Progressive or unresolved feeding difficulties
Asymmetry of muscle tone
Hypotonia or hypertonia
Failure to reach milestones appropriate for "corrected age"

Patient Outcome
Infant will reach his/her physical potential without further compromise to respiratory status.

Nursing Interventions	Rationales
Assess/document neuromuscular exam at each visit; include the respiratory, rest, and sleep status of infant at time of exam.	
Involve developmental therapist in infant's evaluation.	A developmental therapist can determine the extent of neurophysical development and propose methods for enhancing development.
Provide/review with parents explanations on infant handling, positioning, and feeding strategies.	To promote correct anatomical position, strength, and development.
Involve physical therapist/occupational therapist and parents in the development of individualized patient strategies.	
Assess parent's implementation of program and their evaluation of infant's progress.	
Make information available for parents about early evaluation and intervention programs appropriate and available for infant.	These programs provide specialized, individualized care and instruction that have proven to be effective in enhancing development in children with special needs and developmental delays.

▼

NURSING DIAGNOSIS: KNOWLEDGE DEFICIT (CAREGIVER) REGARDING SKILLS NECESSARY IN CARE OF CHRONICALLY, OFTEN PROGRESSIVELY ILL INFANT

Related To
- Lack of exposure
- Unfamiliarity with information resources

Defining Characteristics
Few or repeated questions
Hesitancy in assuming care
Inaccurate follow-through of instructions

Patient Outcome
Parents acknowledge confidence, reliability, and readiness in assuming all care needs of their infant.

Nursing Interventions	Rationales
Determine parental readiness and involvement in assuming new responsibilities. Assess competency and confidence of parental care actions.	Ideally, the ambulatory care nurse has become acquainted with the family prior to the infant's discharge home and has developed a rapport with them as she has been involved with the development of the home care plan.
Review discharge plan with parents/caregivers; provide ongoing education regarding care needs.	Ongoing planning and coordination of care is essential. Renegotiations of care plans must be made to suit the needs of the infant and family at home. This may require modification of the discharge plan but must be done with careful instruction and documentation in collaboration with the pediatrician and/or pulmonary specialist.
Anticipate possible care needs that may arise so that discussions, questions, and instruction may be established prior to actual need for implementation.	
Foster self-esteem in caregivers with praise and by allowing them to provide for infant's care needs.	This instills confidence that they *can* handle child's care needs.

▼

NURSING DIAGNOSIS: HIGH RISK FOR INEFFECTIVE FAMILY COPING

Risk Factors
- Compromised "sick" family member
- Time-consuming care needs of one member

- Unresolved guilt over premature birth with its sequelae
- Alterations in parenting efforts

Patient Outcomes

Needs of each family member and of the family unit will be met without undue stress.

Nursing Interventions	Rationales
Assess family dynamics.	The infant's need for intensive care, and often long-term or recurrent hospitalizations, may have deprived family of normal interactions and attachments during the crucial neonatal period. In addition, BPD infants often have difficult temperaments and behavioral patterns that may be time consuming and, as the infant grows, may be a source of frustration and manipulation in the family.
Assess growth and development of all children.	Parents may assume overprotective or over-indulgent behavior with siblings; they may avoid or be unable to address emotional and physical needs of other children.
Assess past/current coping skills of parents and family.	Individuals with history/pattern of unsuccessful coping may need additional resources.
Observe family unit in care of infant during visit and in home if possible.	
Coordinate appointments, visits with all medical team members so that limited time is necessary for follow-up visits.	Wasted time during scheduled appointments/unnecessary visits promote noncompliance.
Ask parents "How is it going?" and *allow time* for observations, questions and answers that give key information to family coping.	Parents may have difficulty expressing fears, concerns, and guilt.
Help family identify and mobilize available support networks.	Caregivers require emotional support and respite care.

▼

DISCHARGE PLANNING/CONTINUITY OF CARE

- Follow up visits with a phone call to assess how plan of care is working in home environment.
- Refer to pediatric and/or pulmonary specialist.
- Provide needed consultation and community referrals for family support.
- Refer to physical therapist/occupational therapist/developmental therapist as needed.

CANDIDIASIS

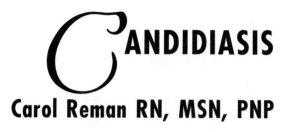

Carol Reman RN, MSN, PNP

Candidiasis is a fungal infection commonly seen in the mouth, (moniliasis or oral thrush), on the skin (dermatitis), or in the vagina (monilial vaginitis). Contributory factors include diabetes, high-dose steroid or antibiotic therapy, malnutrition, and poor hygiene allowing overgrowth of the candida normally present in the gastrointestinal tract and vagina. Infants have no immune factor to *Candida* until approximately 6 months of age, and therefore may become infected during descent through the birth canal.

ETIOLOGY

Fungal organism *Candida albicans*

CLINICAL MANIFESTATIONS

Mouth
- Cheesy white plaques along buccal mucosa, gums, and tongue, that can't be wiped away
- May or may not cause discomfort

Skin
- Beefy red, shiny maculopapular lesions, commonly seen in diaper area
- Satellite lesions around affected area
- Causes discomfort when skin is wet

Vagina
- Cheesy white plaque along vagina
- Vaginal discharge
- Itching

CLINICAL/DIAGNOSTIC FINDINGS

Positive culture for *Candida*

▼

NURSING DIAGNOSIS: IMPAIRED SKIN INTEGRITY

Related To
- Chemical substances (sensitivity to diaper products/detergents)
- Hyperthermia (body heat and moisture)
- Poor hygiene

Defining Characteristics

Disruption of skin surface
Pain
Inability to eat or drink
Irritability

Patient Outcomes

- The child's infected area will be lesion free.
- The child
  – will tolerate food and fluids.
  – will not experience reinfection.

Nursing Interventions	Rationales
Assess for presence of lesions.	All sites of infection must be identified and effectively treated to prevent recurrence.
Determine causative/contributing factors:	
1. hygiene practices	Poor handwashing techniques, not changing diapers frequently
2. change in diaper products	Allergic response
3. antibiotic therapy	Reduces natural protective organisms.
4. condition of mother's nipples, if breast-feeding	Broken, irritated skin on the breast-feeding mother's nipples increases the risk of contracting a candidiasis from the infant. The mother may have an infection and will reinfect the infant if breast infection remains untreated.

Nursing Interventions	Rationales
For diaper/skin dermatitis, instruct to	
1. change diaper frequently.	Moisture promotes fungal growth.
2. expose area to air several times during day.	
3. apply topical Mycostatin cream or Lotrimin Cream 1% four times daily until rash disappears.	
4. avoid nonprescribed powders and creams.	These can coat skin, hold in moisture, and promote fungal growth.
For oral lesions	
1. treat with Nystatin oral suspension (1 mL) to each side of mouth four times daily, *after meals.*	
2. instruct in good oral hygiene: baby's mouth, cleaning baby bottles, nipples.	
3. if breast-feeding mother has red, tender nipples, instruct to coat with Nystatin cream/suspension four times daily.	The mother also must be treated to prevent reinfection in the child.
For vaginitis	
1. apply miconazole nitrate (Monistat) cream as prescribed.	
2. use Nystatin vaginal suppository as preferred.	
3. instruct in need to take medication for prescribed time (usually 14 days).	The fungal infection will *not* be suppressed and can recur easily with suboptimal therapy.
4. Keep underpants clean and dry.	Moisture and heat promote fungal growth.

▼

NURSING DIAGNOSIS: PAIN

Related To
- Skin lesions
- Mucous membrane lesions
- Inflamed tissue

Defining Characteristics

Facial mask of pain
Restlessness
Crying after urination
Difficulty eating/drinking
Vaginal itching

Patient Outcomes

The child will
- be able to eat and drink without difficulty.
- appear comfortable.
- verbalize cessation of pain/discomfort/itching.

Nursing Interventions	Rationales
Assess source and degree of pain.	Oral thrush may or may not cause discomfort; vaginal itching/diaper rash can be quite uncomfortable.
For oral lesions 1. assess child's ability to eat and drink.	Open oral lesions can be painful and inhibit adequate nutritional intake.
2. instruct parent on use of oral topical analgesic before feedings.	Topical oral analgesia may be necessary to relieve pain and thereby to prevent dehydration. Response should be almost immediate.
3. offer foods/fluids that are nonacidic and soft.	

Nursing Interventions	Rationales
For diaper rash, instruct to 1. apply topical antifungal ointment. 2. keep area clean and dry; change diaper frequently. 3. remove diaper whenever possible. 4. apply 1% hydrocortisone cream for severe erythema.	
For vaginal itching, instruct to apply Mycolog cream to affected area.	

▼

DISCHARGE PLANNING/CONTINUITY OF CARE

- Request child be seen in 4–5 days if no improvements. Consider immunology consult for recurrent lesions.
- LaLeche League will provide mother with breast care information, or refer to breast-feeding consultant.
- Obtain gynecological consult for child/adolescent with vaginitis.

$\mathcal{C}$HICKEN POX (VARICELLA)

Michele Knoll Puzas, RNC, MHPE

Chicken pox is a communicable disease transmitted primarily through respiratory droplet spread and secondarily by direct contact with weeping lesions. Respiratory secretions are contagious before the outbreak of skin lesions. Crusted vesicles are no longer contagious. Incubation is approximately 14 days but can be up to 21 days.

ETIOLOGIES

- Virus—varicella zoster (V-Z)
- Immunization not yet available

CLINICAL MANIFESTATIONS

- Child appears ill before rash appears: low-grade fever, irritability, anorexia, and malaise.
- As rash appears, prodromal symptoms diminish, usually in 24 hr.
- Rash begins on trunk, usually in covered areas and creases, then spreads outward to face, upper arms, and legs.
- Rash is highly pruritic, and develops from macule to papule to vesicle in rapid sequence. Vesicles break easily, weep slightly, and crust over. All stages can be seen at one time over the child's body.

CLINICAL/DIAGNOSTIC FINDINGS

None required

▼

NURSING DIAGNOSIS: INFECTION

Related To
- Contact with contagious person
- Varicella zoster virus

90

Defining Characteristics

Fever
Lymphadenopathy
Malaise
Anorexia
Irritability
Rash

Patient Outcomes

Child will be isolated from general social contact during period of communicability.

Nursing Interventions	Rationales
Assess for history of exposure.	Helps confirm diagnosis in early stage.
Assess acuity of illness and determine presence of complications:	Child who is immunosuppressed or presents with complications may require hospitalization.
1. Observe skin for evidence of secondary bacterial infection. 2. Evaluate neurological status.	
3. Evaluate respiratory function.	Encephalitis and V-Z pneumonia can be life threatening; complications are rare.
Discuss period of communicability with parents. Inform parents that 1. child must be isolated from high-risk individuals (newborns, immunosuppressed). 2. child should stay home from school/day care for about 1 week to 10 days.	Most vesicles are dried/crusted in about 7 days after onset.

▼

NURSING DIAGNOSIS: PAIN

Related To infection/rash/lymphadenopathy

Defining Characteristics

Generalized malaise
Pruritis
Complaint of discomfort
Restlessness

Patient Outcome

The child will verbalize less itching, increased comfort.

Nursing Interventions	Rationales
Determine extent of rash and presence of secondary infections.	Some children experience only minor rash outbreak and are less uncomfortable than those with extensive rash. Secondary infection will cause more pain at the site.
Instruct parent to 1. apply calamine lotion to rash; dot infected lesions with antimicrobial ointment.	
2. allow child to take warm water baths (baking soda or Aveeno may be added to bath).	Baths significantly lessen pruritis.
3. administer acetaminophen for fever and lymphadenopathy.	
4. avoid giving children aspirin products.	Aspirin use in children with viral illness has been associated with increased risk of developing Reye's Syndrome. Aspirin also may contribute to thrombocytopenia seen occasionally with V-Z infection.
5. administer Benadryl (diphenhydramine hydrochloride) or antihistamine.	This helps to control itching. These medications can make the child sleepy or hyperactive and should be used sparingly.
6. keep child's hands clean and fingernails short; apply mittens if needed.	This is to lessen scratching and risk of scarring.
7. provide diversional activities.	
8. explain to child that scratching can cause infection and scarring.	
9. provide warm saline solution or diluted hydrogen peroxide for oral rinses.	This helps to alleviate pain caused by oral lesions.

Nursing Interventions	Rationales
Explain to parent that disease is self-limiting and child will be immune from reoccurrence.	

▼

DISCHARGE PLANNING/CONTINUITY OF CARE

- Follow-up is not necessary unless signs of complications develop.
- Refer infants, high-risk children to immunologist.
- Arrange hospitalization if needed.

CHILD ABUSE/NEGLECT

Cathleen Kiely, RN, BSN

Child abuse/neglect refers to the physical, psychological, or sexual abuse and/or neglect of a child. The nurse sees children in a variety of settings (school, clinic, physician's office, emergency room) and always should be sensitive to potential injury as well as cause for actual injuries presented.

ETIOLOGIES

- Lack of understanding of normal child development
- Lack of social-economic support
- Lack of parental attachment
- Parent's own unmet parenting needs
- Psychological disorder
- Overwhelming stress

CLINICAL MANIFESTATIONS

See Nursing Diagnosis: Potential or Actual Injury, Defining Characteristics

CLINICAL/DIAGNOSTIC FINDINGS

- Positive cultures
- Positive x-rays

▼

NURSING DIAGNOSIS: POTENTIAL OR ACTUAL INJURY

Related To
- Physical abuse/neglect
- Sexual abuse

Defining Characteristics
Actual
- Fractures
  - spiral
  - multiple fractures in various stages of healing

- Burns
  - absence of splash marks
  - on soles of feet, palms of hands, back or buttocks
  - symmetrical burns
  - pattern descriptive of object used
- Bruises/welts
  - various stages of healing
  - pattern descriptive of object used
- Poisoning as a result of lack of supervision: drug overdose
- Sexually transmitted diseases
- Lacerations or bruises to external genitalia

Potential
- Torn, bloody, stained underclothing
- Poor medical follow-up (i.e., missed appointments, immunizations not up to date)
- Any child given inappropriate food/drink
- Uncleanliness

Nursing Interventions	Rationales
Obtain history from caregiver and child in nonthreatening manner.	Provides conducive approach to enhance willingness to respond.
Assess for actual injuries: 1. Assess for head injury, respiratory distress, and level of consciousness. Provide emergent care as necessary to preserve airway, breathing, and circulation. 2. Assess extremity(s) for fracture, including movement, circulation, and sensation. Maintain body in functional alignment. 3. Assess size, depth, color, and location of wounds. Assess wound for redness, swelling, or drainage. Cleanse wounds. 4. Assess for potential sexual abuse: • laceration, bruises to external genitalia • complaints of pain on urination/defecation • blood in urine or stool.	

Nursing Interventions	Rationales
Assess relationship between child and caregiver.	This may help confirm suspicion of abusive relationships. Often, however, such interactions may seem appropriate while child and caregiver are in the doctor's office.
Document all assessments (using drawings as applicable).	This is necessary for comparison on serial exam. The medical record is a legal document; accurate documentation is necessary if it is to be used as such.
If child's physical condition warrants, facilitate transportation to emergency room or inpatient unit as applicable.	

▼

NURSING DIAGNOSIS: ALTERED NUTRITION—LESS THAN BODY REQUIREMENTS

Related To
• Physical neglect
• Inadequate intake

Defining Characteristics
Poor weight gain
Lack of tears
Poor skin turgor
Sunken eyes
Constipation/diarrhea

Patient Outcomes
Child will maintain
• recommended body weight
• adequate fluid and electrolyte balance

Nursing Interventions	Rationales
Assess weight every office/clinic visit and document.	This is for future comparison.

Nursing Interventions	Rationales
Obtain nutritional history: 1. type of formula/food 2. amount of formula/food 3. frequency of meals 4. tolerance	Information is necessary to distinguish between food intolerance and improper feeding.
Assess gastrointestinal status: 1. bowel movement 2. frequency 3. consistency 4. nausea or vomiting	This is necessary to rule out organic/physical disorder.
Provide clearly written and concise feeding schedules.	
Instruct caregiver on use of feeding diary.	This helps in determining differential diagnosis.
Obtain social work consult.	This assists in determining if problem is related to social, economic, or psychological status.
Initiate intravenous hydration and hospitalization if needed.	

▼

NURSING DIAGNOSIS: ALTERED PARENTING

Related To
- Poor parenting role models
- Low maturation level of parent
- Lack of support
- Situational crises

Defining Characteristics
Demonstrates lack of concern, detachment, or overreaction to child's injury
Does not accompany child on office visit
Verbalizes or demonstrates inappropriate expectations of child
Perceives child as being a special problem
Verbalizes lack of parenting skills, inadequate coping skills, lack of control, or feelings of inadequacy

Patient Outcome
Parent/caregiver will verbalize and demonstrate appropriate parenting skills.

Nursing Interventions	Rationales
Observe parent-child conversations, play, and interaction.	
Assess for factors that contribute to parenting difficulties: 1. cultural and socioeconomic status 2. low educational/maturation level of parent 3. poor family/support structure 4. minimal knowledge regarding child development.	Presence of risk factors along with physical evidence requires further investigation to protect the child.
Refer parent/caregiver to social services agency for enrollment in parenting skills class.	Groups that come together for mutual support/information can be helpful.
Provide written material on appropriate growth and development of the child, if needed.	
Demonstrate appropriate conversations/play/actions with child.	Parent may learn better through observation.
Inform parents of all concerns regarding suspected abuse/neglect.	
Allow parent to verbalize concerns regarding child's physical, psychological, or sexual abuse/neglect status.	Parent may or may not be aware that abuse or neglect has occurred. Encouraging open communication allows for identification of educational needs versus psychosocial needs.
Inform parent that, because of the nature of the child's injuries and/or potential risk to child's health, proper authorities will be notified and the home environment/family will be evaluated.	

▼

NURSING DIAGNOSIS: SELF-ESTEEM DISTURBANCE (CHILD)

Related To
- Psychological neglect/abuse
- Sexual abuse
- Physical abuse/neglect

Defining Characteristics
Destructive/hostile
Self-abuse or self-negating verbalizations
Withdrawn/passive
Change in behavior
Expressions of guilt or shame
Excessive masturbation
Sleep disturbance
Suicide attempts
Substance abuse

Patient Outcome
Child will begin to verbalize/demonstrate positive feelings about self.

Nursing Interventions	Rationales
Assess interactions between child and parent and staff. Assess child's ability to interact with those around him/her, and the degree of spontaneity in these interactions.	Provides information on the child's comfort level in social settings. Abused children may be withdrawn.
Assess child's perception of self.	Most abused children suffer from low self-esteem and distorted sense of their qualities as a person.
Assess coping mechanism (see Defining Characteristics)	
Provide calm, reassuring environment.	Most children have difficulty acknowledging and/or verbalizing feelings.
Structure appropriate coping mechanisms, including verbal and nonverbal outlets. 1. Acknowledge feelings verbalized by child. 2. Reflect back to feelings verbalized. 3. Provide nonverbal outlets for expression: • paper and crayons, writing paper/pens. • dolls.	This is to validate understanding of feelings.
Provide feedback about child's strengths.	Feedback will increase his/her self-awareness and insight.

Nursing Interventions	Rationales
Remind child that he/she is no way responsible for abuse.	
Explore availability of support groups or programs.	

▼

DISCHARGE PLANNING/CONTINUITY OF CARE

- Follow up based on physical injuries/illness.
- Obtain consults:
  - social work
  - nutrition
  - psychiatric
  - play therapy
- Refer parents to self-help organization, if available.
- Notify appropriate local authority if abuse or neglect is suspected.

$\mathcal{C}$HLAMYDIA

Jeffrey Zurlinden, RN, MS

Chlamydia is a sexually transmitted disease that is becoming more common in sexually active adolescents. It causes a localized infection of the urethra, endocervical canal, rectum, or pharynx. The patient may have one site of infection or many sites. The infection is spread by sexual contact with the infected site. Untreated infections may lead to pelvic inflammatory disease (PID) and reproductive difficulties as a result of scarring. Infection in the young child may indicate sexual abuse.

ETIOLOGY

Infection with bacteria *Chlamydia trachomatis*

CLINICAL MANIFESTATIONS

- Asymptomatic
- Yellowish discharge
- Dysuria
- Spotting between menstrual periods
- Rectal itching
- Changes in bowel habits
- Blood or mucus in stools
- Scant, mucoid penile discharge

CLINICAL/DIAGNOSTIC FINDINGS

Positive cultures or enzyme-linked immunosorbent assays (ELISA)

▼

NURSING DIAGNOSIS: INFECTION

Related To presence of infectious organisms

Defining Characteristics

Positive tissue culture from urethra, endocervical canal, throat, or rectum

Gram's stain with polymorphonuclear leukocytes and no gram-negative intracellular diplococci on smear

Positive chlamydia ELISA result from endocervical, urethral, or throat specimens

Persistent symptoms despite treatment for gonorrhea (GC) and negative GC cultures

History of sexual contact with an infected person

Patient Outcome

Patient will exhibit no signs of infection, as evidenced by resolution of discharge, and negative cultures.

Nursing Interventions	Rationales
Check local and state regulations to determine if sexually transmitted diseases (STDs) are reportable to the health department.	
Determine date of last sexual contact, number of sexual partners, and description of recent sexual activities.	This provides information regarding behaviors that increases risk of STDs.
Obtain cultures from all sites of possible infection.	Patients may present with multiple sites of infection.
Obtain smears from discharges.	
Obtain history of previous STDs.	Although chlamydial infections are easily cured with antibiotics, they do tend to recur.
Assess 1. Urethral or cervical discharge. 2. Urinary frequency. 3. Pain or burning when urinating. 4. Spotting between menstrual periods or after intercourse. 5. Rectal discharge. 6. Mucus or blood in stools. 7. Rectal spasms. 8. Change in bowel movements.	Eight percent of women are asymptomatic. If symptomatic, mucoid yellowish discharge, less profuse than with GC, occurs within 21 days after infection.
Screen for other STDs, hepatitis B, and human immunodeficiency virus (HIV).	Patients with one STD are at higher risk for a concomitant STD.

Nursing Interventions	**Rationales**
For women, obtain menstrual history, including date of last period.	It can be difficult to get cultures during menstruation; results are less accurate (increased number of false negatives), especially with tampon use.
Determine method of and compliance with birth control.	Contracting STDs suggests no use/improper use of condoms. Adolescents are at especially high risk for pregnancy. Nurse should use this opportunity for health screening/education.
Check local and state regulations to determine if minors can receive abortions or birth control counseling without parental notification or consent.	
Perform pregnancy test.	This is necessary for early detection of pregnancy. Young women can become pregnant before menarche, and some drugs have teratogenic effect. Tetracycline is contraindicated for use with pregnant women.
Check local and state regulations to determine if minors can receive treatment for STDs without parental notification or consent.	
Administer antibiotics as ordered.	Treatment for chlamydia frequently changes in response to the development of new antibiotics. Usually doxycycline, tetracycline, azithromycin, or ofloxacin is used. Follow the current guidelines from the Centers for Disease Control (CDC) or local Health Department.
Observe for possible anaphylactic reaction to intramuscular antibiotics given during clinic visit.	

Nursing Interventions	Rationales
Dispense condoms.	The use of latex condoms is the most effective means of preventing the spread of disease during sexual contact.
Instruct patient to inform all recent sexual partners (within the last 3 weeks) of possible exposure to chlamydia and need for treatment.	Untreated asymptomatic sexual partners are common source of reinfection.
Determine if sexual contact was consensual. Refer to social services if sexual abuse is suspected.	

▼

NURSING DIAGNOSIS: KNOWLEDGE DEFICIT

Related To new diagnosis

Defining Characteristics
Patient asks many questions
Patient asks few questions
Patient has history of repeated infections
Patient is unable to state the causes, treatment, and prevention of chlamydia

Patient Outcomes
Patient will state
- medication schedule.
- medication side effects.
- date of return visits for test of cure.
- how to use condoms to prevent future infections.

Nursing Interventions	Rationales
Assess patient's present level of understanding.	Misconceptions can increase anxiety/fear and foster spread of STDs.
Instruct about medication schedule and side effects of antibiotics used to treat chlamydia.	Treatment for chlamydia frequently changes in response to new antibiotics. Follow the current guidelines from the CDC or your local Health Department.

Nursing Interventions	Rationales
Instruct on mode of transmission: local inoculation of bacteria from penis to throat, vagina, or rectum.	
Instruct patient to use latex condoms or use other nonintercourse sexual methods to prevent future infections.	Latex condoms are an effective barrier against contact with chancres.
Inform patient of the possible consequences of untreated chlamydia.	PID or difficulty conceiving as a result of scarred fallopian tubes are common complications.

▼

NURSING DIAGNOSIS: INEFFECTIVE MANAGEMENT OF THERAPEUTIC REGIMEN

Related To
- Unwillingness to comply with treatment, prevention, or informing sexual partners
- Complexity of treatment regimen

Defining Characteristics
Persistent infection not caused by antibiotic-resistant strains
Missed return visits for test of cure
Incorrect pill count at return visit
Inadequate blood level of antibiotic

Patient Outcomes
Patient will
- complete course of treatment.
- notify sexual partners.
- use condoms to prevent infection.

Nursing Interventions	Rationales
Compare actual effect and expected therapeutic effect.	
Plot patient's pattern of returning for follow-up visits.	
Determine social support systems and presence of significant others.	Interpersonal influences can impact on compliance with treatment regimen.

Nursing Interventions	Rationales
Assess patient's and significant other's beliefs about current illness and treatment plan.	How one perceives susceptibility, severity, and threat of disease impacts on health behaviors.
Assess quality of relationship between patient and health care workers and health care facility.	
Role play to practice informing sexual partners of possible exposure to chlamydia.	This gives patient an opportunity to rehearse situations and allows nurse to provide feedback.
Suggest short-term therapy, if patient has a history of not taking oral medication.	Less complex therapies facilitate compliance. Azithromycin is a single dose.
Role play to practice new behaviors in situations leading to reinfection (such as saying "no" or using condoms).	
Develop a positive relationship with the patient that encourages participation with treatment decisions.	The nurse-patient relationship is based on recognition of patient's right to self-determination and capacity for self-management, with focus on decision making and goal attainment.
Determine with the patient the plan of treatment she is most likely to complete.	Involving the patient in planning the regimen improves compliance.

▼

NURSING DIAGNOSIS: ALTERED SEXUALITY PATTERNS

Related To
- Imposed restrictions
- Fear
- Risk of contagion

Defining Characteristics
Patient or significant other expresses concern about the effects chlamydia and treatment have on their expressions of physical intimacy.

Patient Outcome
Patient will state ways of expressing physical intimacy during treatment.

Nursing Interventions	Rationales
Determine patient's or significant other's concerns.	STD diagnosis may provoke feelings of guilt, shame, the need for punishment, or other anxiety-provoking thoughts unique to the patient.
Determine if concerns also are related to fears about acquired immunodeficiency syndrome (AIDS).	An STD diagnosis may provoke fear of AIDS that alters sexual behavior.
Assess perception of meaning of chlamydia infection.	Provides opportunity to correct misconceptions.
Elicit patient's feeling about limits on sexual behavior.	
Interview patient in a quiet, private, distraction-free environment.	Most women are hesitant to discuss personal sexual matters. The proper setting may facilitate discussion.
Explore ways to express physical intimacy during treatment excluding vaginal, rectal, and pharyngeal intercourse.	Restrictions on sexual activity should not deprive the couple of other activities that convey the message that they are loved and desired.
Explore ways to express physical intimacy that do not lead to reinfection.	Barrier contraception with latex condoms is effective.

▼

DISCHARGE PLANNING/CONTINUITY OF CARE

- Arrange gynecology consult.
- Instruct patient to return for routine screening if high-risk sexual behavior continues.
- Instruct patient to report persistence or recurrence of symptoms.
- Refer for HIV counseling and testing.
- Refer to family planning clinic.

*C*OLIC

Alison Benzies Miklos, RNC, MSN
Dawn E. Reimann, RN, MS

Infantile colic, also known as irritable infant syndrome, is a paroxysmal abdominal pain of intestinal origin accompanied by persistent and inconsolable crying.

ETIOLOGIES

Unknown. Possibilities include:
- immaturity of the infant's gastrointestinal tract and nervous system
- excessive gas production
- sensitivity to cow's milk protein
- lactose malabsorption
- improper feeding techniques
- emotional stress between parent and child

CLINICAL MANIFESTATIONS

- Emerges by second week of life
- Persists until 6 months of age
- Usually ends by 12 weeks of age
- Rhythmic attacks of screaming
- Increased motor activity
- Disrupted feeding and sleeping patterns

CLINICAL/DIAGNOSTIC FINDINGS

None

▼

NURSING DIAGNOSIS: PAIN

Related To paroxysmal abdominal spasms

Defining Characteristics
Persistent crying without obvious cause
Inconsolable
Clenched fists, arched back
Face red, flushed
Abdomen tense, possibly distended
Sucks vigorously, then rejects nipple
May seem to have excessive gas

Patient Outcomes
The child will
• appear comfortable.
• have decreased crying episodes.

Nursing Interventions	Rationales
Obtain a thorough history of the infant's usual daily events: 1. diet 2. time of day when attacks occur 3. relationship of attacks to feedings 4. number of bowel movements associated with symptoms.	Attacks frequently occur at a specific time of day. By determining the events that possibly contribute to the onset of the attack, the parent may be able to manipulate those events or environmental conditions that precipitate the attack. Bowel movements are normal in colic; however, constipation, blood, or mucus in the stool may suggest other intestinal problems (e.g., obstruction, infection).
Assess infant's behavior and his/her response to stimuli (e.g., persistent crying, excessive flatus, inconsolable).	
Encourage parents to administer 1–2 oz of warm water.	
Place infant in prone position over a covered hot water bottle or heated, rolled towel.	Warmth helps stimulate peristalsis and relieve abdominal cramping.
Insert the bulb of a rectal thermometer into the rectum.	Stimulates passage of flatus and feces.

Nursing Interventions	Rationales

Instruct parents on calming techniques for relief of colic:
1. Change infant's position frequently.
2. Massage abdomen.
3. Walk with infant, face down, with his/her body across parent's arm and hand under abdomen, gently applying pressure.
4. Provide vestibular motion with white noise, such as:
  • rocking
  • car rides
  • radio static
  • sound of vacuum cleaner
  • walking
  • bouncing motion
  • place in wind-up swing
  • use commercial devices (e.g. car ride simulators and recordings of womb sounds)
5. Reduce sensory stimulation:
  • dim lights
  • swaddle
  • avoid loud noises
	Rhythmic sound and movement alleviates tension.

Instruct parents to 1. provide pacifier for nonnutritive sucking. 2. offer glucose water.	Glucose water or a pacifier may help increase peristalsis, thereby moving intestinal gas through the intestines to relieve pain.
Instruct parents in techniques for administration of medications, if ordered, (e.g., sedatives, anticholinergics, antispasmodics, antiflatulents).	
Obtain a 24-hr dietary history in the lactating mother. Encourage mother to eliminate gas-producing foods from her diet.	Reinforce that gas-producing foods such as vegetables, spices, caffeine products, and chocolate may cause gas and discomfort in the infant.
Suggest mother eliminate cow's milk products from her diet for 5 days.	Milk products, ingested by the mother, pass through breast milk and may precipitate colic in the infant who has a sensitivity to cow's milk products.

Nursing Interventions	Rationales
Observe feeding procedure. Encourage smaller, frequent feedings.	Increased carbohydrate ingestion or overfeeding may lead to excess fermentation and gas production. Smaller feedings help prevent distention.
Burp infant during and after feeding with infant upright over shoulder. Place infant in an upright position after feedings.	Improper bottle position and/or inadequate burping may result in excessive air ingestion causing gas accumulation. Upright positions help air bubbles rise.
Discuss the use of collapsible feeding bags in bottles.	Collapsible feeding bags decrease air ingestion.

▼

NURSING DIAGNOSIS: INEFFECTIVE COPING (PARENTS)

Related To
- Situational crisis (infant with colic)
- Inadequate support system/resources
- Unrealistic perceptions
- Inadequate coping method

Defining Characteristics
Verbalization of inability to cope
Inability to meet role expectations as parent
Emotional tension
Inability to problem solve
Frustration
Frequent phone calls to the pediatrician's office
Loss of control
Parental crying
Fatigue
Depression
Helplessness
Anxiety

Patient Outcome
Parent's verbal responses and actions indicate positive feelings toward infant.

Nursing Interventions	Rationales
Assess parent's knowledge of colic.	
Educate parents on what is known about colic (e.g., etiology, the common characteristics, the duration of colic). Educate parents on normal infant crying behavior.	Infants average $1\frac{1}{2}$–4 hr of crying daily in the first several weeks of life. At about 6–8 weeks, crying begins to decrease.
Discuss the infant's well-being.	Infants with colic do gain weight and tolerate their feedings.
Assess parental response to colic attacks and the methods utilized to relieve infant's crying.	
Inform parents that their responses of anxiety and tension may increase the infant's irritability, tension, and crying.	
Inform parents that letting their infant cry for a short period of time (15–20 min) will allow the infant to try self-consoling techniques such as sucking on a finger. Instruct parents not to allow the infant to cry for longer than 20 min.	Giving parents permission to let their infants cry may help decrease parental anxiety and family tension, which may result in a calmer infant. The longer and more intense the crying becomes the more difficult it is to calm the infant.
Reinforce the fact that the condition of colic is temporary.	It usually lessens after 3–4 months of age and is a time-limited problem.
Evaluate parental coping mechanisms in dealing with infantile colic.	Colicky infants often create a sense of emotional instability in parents. These feelings could lead to occurrences of child abuse (e.g., shaking syndrome.)
Encourage parents to arrange for respite time, especially when they are tired or anxious.	Suggest the use of support systems and allow others to care for the infant.
Caution parents against shaking their infant.	Shaking the infant may cause damage to cerebral vessels and vertebrae of the neck.
Reassure parents that negative feelings toward the infant and feelings of inadequate parenting are normal.	

DISCHARGE PLANNING/CONTINUITY OF CARE

- Assure parents that they can call their health care provider for further help or suggestions in managing their infant.
- Follow up at routine infant exam.
- Make referrals as needed:
  - psychotherapeutic counseling
  - social service
  - LaLeche League

CONJUNCTIVITIS

Barbara Ruth Bellar, PAC

Conjunctivitis (pink eye, red eye, hyperemia) is the irritation of the conjunctiva of one or both eyes, causing photophobia, itching, burning, swelling and depending on the cause, purulent discharge.

ETIOLOGIES

- Infections—viral or bacterial
- Allergic reaction
- Trauma
- Secondary to systemic disorder

CLINICAL MANIFESTATIONS

- Hyperemia—diffuse redness of sclera
- Conjunctival inflammation—diffuse redness of the mucous membrane that lines the inner eyelids and covers the sclera

CLINICAL/DIAGNOSTIC FINDINGS

Positive culture (bacterial)

▼

NURSING DIAGNOSIS: INFECTION

Related To
- Adenovirus
- Herpes simplex
- *Staphylococcus*
- *Pneumococcus*

- *Haemophilus*
- *Moraxella*

Defining Characteristics

Viral
Gradual onset
Copious tearing
Minimal itching
Exudate
Occasional blurring of vision
Swollen preauricular nodes, usually unilateral
Generalized hyperemia
Mild photophobia

Bacterial
Sudden onset
Tearing
Burning
Minimal itching
Generalized hyperemia
Profuse purulent exudate
Associated with sore throat and fever

Patient Outcomes

- The child will display no signs of infection, as evidenced by clear white sclera and absence of itching and burning.
- The child's vision will be within normal limits.

Nursing Interventions	Rationales
Assess gross appearance of sclera and conjunctiva. Observe for discharge.	A pseudomembrane may be visualized with a bacterial infection.
Perform Snellen chart exam—appropriate to age. Inform parent of any decreased visual acuity.	Visual acuity will need to be re-evaluated once illness is controlled. Corrective lenses may be needed.
Assess pupil reactions in darkened room. Assess fundi of each eye.	
Palpate preauricular nodes for enlargement or tenderness.	
Explain viral conjunctivitis. Assure that condition will clear up in 5–14 days.	Hyperemia is caused by local relaxation of arterioles and will resolve when virus is gone.

Nursing Interventions	Rationales
Explain that bacterial infection is extremely contagious. Obtain smear for culture if needed.	
Instruct on 1. proper handwashing. 2. application of moist compress to remove exudate. 3. instillation of eyedrops/ ointment.	Antimicrobial treatment can lessen duration and severity of symptoms. Most causative organisms are Gram positive, therefore, erythromycin, gentamycin, tobramycin, or sulfacetamide may be ordered.

▼

NURSING DIAGNOSIS: ALTERED SKIN INTEGRITY

Related To
- Presence of foreign body
- Trauma
- Allergic response
- Systemic disease

Defining Characteristics

Trauma/foreign body
Sudden onset
Unilateral or bilateral local redness
Tearing
Pain
Sensation of particle on eye surface
Vision normal except in case of major trauma

Allergic
Severe itching
Generalized hyperemia
Moderate tearing
Mucous exudate
Gradual onset
Bilateral
Rhinorrhea
Conjunctival edema

Systemic
May present as infectious, allergic, or traumatic

Patient Outcomes
- The child's sclera and conjunctiva will be normal in color.
- The child will be relieved of itching, burning, and pain.

Nursing Interventions	Rationales
Perform initial eye exam as previously described.	
Refer for immediate attention in hospital/emergency room if major trauma is observed.	Surgical intervention may be needed; delays could jeopardize vision.
Assess for foreign body: evert upper eyelid, retract lower eyelid and view for grossly apparent foreign body.	
Remove foreign body gently with saline flush and cotton swab.	
Instill antibiotic ointment or solution after foreign body is removed.	
Patch eye and instruct parents to return in 24 hr for re-check.	The eye must be reevaluated for infection/structural damage.
Refer to ophthalmologist if foreign body cannot be removed.	The ophthalmologist will be better able to visualize foreign body and eye trauma requiring intervention.
Assess for allergic response.	
Apply cool compress over eyes and nose.	This promotes vasoconstriction.
Instruct in the use of oral antihistamines and the instillation of eye drops (weak vasoconstrictor or corticosteroid).	Occasionally helpful in controlling symptoms of allergic response.
Advise patients who wear contact lenses to discontinue use temporarily and to consider using preservative-free lens solutions.	Preservatives in some lens solutions have caused allergic hypersensitivity reactions.

▼

DISCHARGE PLANNING/CONTINUITY OF CARE

- Set up follow-up exam for 2 weeks.
- Instruct parent to bring child in sooner if symptoms worsen or for lack of improvement.
- Provide referrals to ophthalmologist.

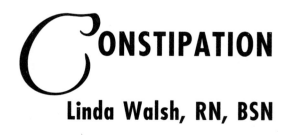

CONSTIPATION

Linda Walsh, RN, BSN

Constipation refers to difficult passage of stool and/or passage of hard stool associated with straining, abdominal pain, or withholding behaviors.

ETIOLOGIES

- Physical
  - poor diet, lack of adequate oral fluids, intolerance of certain infant formulas
  - severe cases could be secondary to bowel obstruction
  - malnutrition
  - cystic fibrosis
- Psychological—anxiety or fear of passage of painful stool
- Developmental—response to dysfunctional approach to toilet training.

CLINICAL MANIFESTATIONS

- Hard, small stool
- Blood-streaked stool
- Abdominal pain or distention
- Less than six bowel movements/week for children < 3 years.
- Less than four bowel movements/week for children > 3 years.
- Anorexia
- Anal fissures—secondary to previous passage of hard stool

CLINICAL/DIAGNOSTIC FINDINGS

None required

▼

NURSING DIAGNOSIS: CONSTIPATION

Related To
- Poor dietary habits
- Fear of pain
- Developmental stage surrounding toilet training

Defining Characteristics
Straining or difficulty in passing stool
Passing of fluid and fecal seepage
Anorexia
Abdominal distention
Nausea and vomiting
Fecal incontinence

Patient Outcomes
Child will
- achieve relief of constipation as evidenced by *regular* passage of soft, formed stool.
- pass stool without pain or associated fear.

Nursing Interventions	Rationales
Assess usual patterns of bowel elimination: type of stool, time of day of evacuation, number of stools per week.	Assessment of problem guides extent/need for treatment.
Assess diet history: usual pattern of eating; amount of fluid intake.	High-fiber foods, fruits and vegetables promote defecation.
Obtain abdominal film if diagnosis is in question.	
Provide caregivers with dietary information: 1. Stress need for adequate fiber and bulk in diet (i.e., vegetables, fruits, juices, whole grains.) 2. Inform that change in infant formula (with or without iron) can precipitate change in bowel habits. 3. Instruct to be alert to food intolerances with introduction of new foods.	

Nursing Interventions	Rationales
Discuss fluid intake. Stress need to take in at least maintenance fluids, including extra water, juices.	
Assess mobility, level of activity.	Activity stimulates gastrointestinal motility.
Explain psychological factors that can affect bowel elimination.	Some children may respond to stressful situations with somatic complaints, including constipation. Toddlers in the process of toilet training might respond with withholding behaviors if pressured. Recommend that toilet training be at child's own pace without punishment for accidents.
Provide quiet, calm environment for evacuation—books, toys, music in the bathroom.	Lack of privacy can worsen constipation.
Discuss medications. Recommend certain over-the-counter preparations for relieving constipation: 1. Colace, Peri-colace (to soften stool) 2. glycerin or Dulcolax 10-mg suppository (soften stool; stimulate rectal mucosa) 3. mineral oil—intestinal lubricant (1 tsp PO A.M.) 4. enema—only when recommended per physician.	Medications should be used only if diet changes have been ineffective.

▼

DISCHARGE PLANNING/CONTINUITY OF CARE

- Request child's primary caregiver to compile log of stool activity: response to laxatives, lubricants.
- Follow up with practitioner on regular basis.
- Refer as needed:
  - nutritionist
  - gastroenterologist/pediatric surgeon
  - psychologist

*C*ROHN'S DISEASE

Audrey Klopp, RN, PhD, ET

Crohn's disease (regional enteritis, inflammatory bowel disease) is an inflammatory bowel disorder that involves all four layers of the portion of the gastrointestinal (GI) tract involved. Crohn's disease may occur anywhere in the GI tract, but most often occurs in the small intestine. Although surgery may be indicated, Crohn's disease typically is managed with steroids, sulfasalazine, and nutritional support. Growth and development typically are delayed as a result of interference in normal nutritional well-being. Crohn's disease may be accompanied by systemic complications, such as arthritis.

ETIOLOGY

Unknown origin

CLINICAL MANIFESTATIONS

- Abdominal pain
- Diarrhea (frequently bloody)
- Weight loss
- Fatigue
- Anorexia
- Onset during preadolescent and adolescent years

CLINICAL/DIAGNOSTIC FINDINGS

- Skip lesions on radiographs or colonoscopy
- Granulomata on biopsy

▼

NURSING DIAGNOSIS: ALTERED NUTRITION—LESS THAN BODY REQUIREMENTS

Related To
- Impaired intestinal absorption
- Anorexia/pain
- Increased nitrogen and fluid loss through diarrhea
- Blood loss from damaged intestinal mucosa

Defining Characteristics

Weight loss
Failure to gain as expected
Small for age
Delayed sexual development
Inadequate intake
Vitamin deficiencies (iron, folate, and zinc)
Dry, scaly skin
Poor skin turgor
Lack of subcutaneous fat
Ridged, clubbed fingernails
Concentrated urine
Fever

Patient Outcomes

- Parent/child will describe foods that are prescribed and those that should be avoided.
- Child will maintain stable body weight.
- Child will maintain normal fluid and electrolyte balance.

Nursing Interventions	Rationales
Teach child/parent about Crohn's disease: 1. typical signs/symptoms 2. usual course of disease 3. possible complications 4. usual treatment/management course and relationship to nutrition.	Crohn's disease is a chronic condition. Impaired absorption causes nutritional abnormalities.
Record child's weight. Assess typical daily intake/output.	During acute episodes, and as disease progresses, weight loss, dehydration, and malnutrition are significant problems.
Assess dietary intolerances.	High-fat, high-residue, and roughage foods aggravate absorption.

Nursing Interventions	Rationales
Assess diarrhea: 1. frequency 2. consistency 3. presence of blood	Accurate assessment aids in detecting potential complications such as dehydration, electrolyte imbalance, and impaired skin integrity.
Assess parent's/child's knowledge of child's specific nutritional needs. Teach child/parent importance of adequate nutrition.	Adequate nutrition is necessary for normal growth and development. Diet management and nutritional support are one of the key treatments in Crohn's disease.
Provide child/parent with nutritional recommendations appropriate to age.	
Modify diet as needed, based on dislikes/intolerances/symptoms as follows: 1. Decrease gas-forming foods. 2. Eliminate "natural laxatives" in children with diarrhea (this includes caffeinated foods/beverages). 3. Reduce fiber if child has stenotic areas of crampy abdominal symptoms. 4. Reduce lactose only if a documented lactose deficiency exists.	Decreases appetite.
Assess parent's financial ability to provide adequate nutrition.	Inability to follow prescribed plan negates achievement of treatment goals. Referrals may be indicated.
Provide vitamin/mineral supplements as prescribed.	This may be required to correct deficiencies. Vitamin B_{12} injections may be required.
Teach parent methods for improving dietary intake, (e.g., allow child to participate in food selection, and preparation of food, avoidance of between-meal snacks).	Giving child some control increases the probability of success.

▼

NURSING DIAGNOSIS: BODY IMAGE DISTURBANCE

Related To
- Side effects of steroids
- Delay in growth and development as compared to peers
- Frequent bouts of diarrhea, pain

Defining Characteristics

Negative verbalization about body appearance and function
Withdrawal from desired or usual activities
Preoccupation with disease
Denial of disease/need for treatment
Crying
Distraction
Complaints of crampy abdominal pain

Patient Outcomes

Child will
- verbalize acceptance of bodily changes.
- speak of self in positive way.

Nursing Interventions	Rationales
Assess child's response to changes in body function and appearance.	Age, developmental stage, family/peer responses can impact on child's view of self.
Assess actual and perceived limitations.	
Encourage child to verbalize fears, concerns, perceived limitations.	Confronting actual/distorted perceptions increases the chance of finding appropriate interventions.
Listen for bowel sounds.	Hyperactive bowel sounds are a typical finding during acute stages of Crohn's disease.
Assess abdominal pain: 1. duration 2. frequency 3. severity—severe abdominal pain may be indicative of perforation 4. relationship to food intake.	Attacks of abdominal pain occur intermittently and subside spontaneously. Frequent bouts of pain negatively impact on body image.

Nursing Interventions	Rationales
Assess child's/parent's perceptions of measures that minimize/relieve abdominal pain. Encourage child/parent to use helpful techniques.	Supporting previously effective interventions can reduce intensity of pain during future bouts. For example, food intolerances, very often individual, may precipitate pain; avoiding these foods may minimize pain.
Teach use of antispasmodic medications and analgesics as prescribed.	
Teach child/parent about additional medications (steroids, sulfasalazine).	Steroids reduce inflammation and suppress the disease. Sulfasalazine is effective for large intestine treatment.
Assess child's/parent's knowledge about expected steroid side effects.	Provides opportunity to clear up misconceptions and prepare child for changes.
Explain expected side effects of steroids; assure child/parent that these side effects abate when steroid therapy is tapered/discontinued.	An understanding of the importance of steroid therapy can improve compliance.
Teach parent/child to use diversional activities in the management of pain.	
Encourage child/parent to focus on strengths and abilities.	Patients with body image disturbance frequently overlook their capabilities and strengths because they are so focused on negative aspects.
Suggest parent/child participate in support group.	Support groups give realistic picture of the disease and ongoing problems/needs/management.

▼

DISCHARGE PLANNING/CONTINUITY OF CARE

- Refer to
  - dietitian
  - mental health professional
  - surgeon
- Encourage child/parent to seek support from peer support group, (e.g., National Colitis and Ileitis Association).

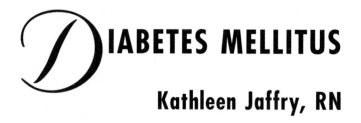

IABETES MELLITUS

Kathleen Jaffry, RN

Diabetes mellitus is a complex disorder of carbohydrate, fat and protein metabolism resulting primarily from a relative or complete lack of insulin secretion by the beta cells of the pancreas. The disease often is familial but may be acquired, as in Cushing's syndrome. The onset of diabetes mellitus is sudden in children, as typically seen in Type I diabetes. Initial presentation will be due to increased thirst, urination, and fatigue. Characteristically the course is progressive. Over time, the eyes, kidneys, nervous system, skin, and circulatory system may be affected; infections are common and atherosclerosis often develops. In childhood, with Type I diabetes when no endogenous insulin is being secreted, ketoacidosis is a constant danger. Ideally, children should be followed by a pediatric endocrinologist.

ETIOLOGIES

- Related to inheritance of certain human leukocyte antigens that predispose an individual to autoimmune destruction of pancreatic islets.
- Viral infection has been suggested as a triggering factor in individuals with a genetic predisposition for diabetes.

CLINICAL MANIFESTATIONS

Major symptoms
- Increased thirst
- Increased urination
- Enuresis
- Increased food ingestion
- Weight loss
- Fatigue
- Hyperglycemia
- Glycosuria

Minor symptoms
- Skin infections
- Dry skin
- Monilial vaginitis in adolescent girls

CLINICAL/DIAGNOSTIC FINDINGS

- Random blood glucose > 200 mg/dL
- Fasting blood glucose > 140 mg/dL

▼

NURSING DIAGNOSIS: ALTERED NUTRITIuN—LESS THAN BODY REQUIREMENTS

Related To inability to absorb nutrients as a result of biological disorder

Defining Characteristics
Weight loss despite increased intake
Weakness
Fatigue

Patient Outcomes
Child will be able to sustain weight within range for age.

Nursing Interventions	Rationales
Obtain weight; compare with standard growth chart.	
Assess for history of weight loss, recent viral illness.	Symptoms of diabetes may not become obvious until the child's body is further stressed by an illness.
Determine usual diet.	This is to determine if improper diet is cause for weight loss or lack of weight gain.
If diet is within normal limits, assess for other signs of diabetes.	
Explain tests necessary to determine diagnosis: 1. urine for glucose/acetone 2. blood for glucose level	

Nursing Interventions	Rationales
Make arrangements for fasting blood glucose and glucose tolerance test.	
If child presents with any signs of ketoacidosis, arrange for immediate hospitalization.	
Arrange referral to endocrinologist and make all further recommendations in collaboration with physician.	

▼

NURSING DIAGNOSIS: INEFFECTIVE INDIVIDUAL COPING

Related To
- Situational crisis
- Unfamiliarity with disease
- Chronic disease

Defining Characteristics
Regressive behavior
Anger/noncompliance with regimen
Refusal to attempt procedures independently
Verbalized inability to cope
Inability to problem solve

Patient Outcome
Child/parent will begin to demonstrate coping behaviors with diabetic condition.

Nursing Interventions	Rationales
Assess patient/parent relationship.	This is to determine parent's ability to support child through crisis.
Assess for noncompliance, anger, regressive behavior in patient.	Child may not be able to verbalize fears/frustrations.
Assess coping mechanisms of patient/parents regarding diagnosis and treatment.	

Nursing Interventions	Rationales
Explain that diabetes can be controlled through diet, insulin, and exercise.	Although diabetes is a life-long, incurable disease, the child can be reassured that control is possible.
Introduce parent and child to peer support groups.	Such groups offer children/teens an alternate means of coping, support, and peer role models.

▼

NURSING DIAGNOSIS: KNOWLEDGE DEFICIT

Related To
- New diagnosis of chronic disease
- Expected life-style changes

Defining Characteristics
Asking many questions
Asking no questions
Noncompliance

Patient Outcomes
Parent and child will be able to
- demonstrate required home care skills.
- state signs/symptoms and treatments of hyper/hypoglycemia.

Nursing Interventions	Rationales
Assess understanding of disease and treatment: hypoglycemia, hyperglycemia, insulin, diet.	This provides baseline for designing teaching plan.
Assess ability to learn, child's developmental level.	Adolescents can assume much more responsibility for self care.
Arrange referral to Certified Diabetes Educator.	
Document progress toward learning goals.	This is an extensive amount of information, knowledge, and skills. Documentation decreases chance of omitting important issues.
Explain the need for insulin, the different types available, and the way to administer it.	

Nursing Interventions	Rationales
Show parent/child how to prepare and mix the insulin.	
Explain need for proper timing of administration.	Proper timing is necessary to prevent hyper and hypoglycemia. Maintaining blood sugar in acceptable range helps prevent complications.
Explain to patient how to home monitor blood sugar and to keep record of blood sugar levels.	This assists the health care team in evaluating management program.
Explain the importance of following proper diet. Explain the four food groups and the exchange list.	Educating child on importance of proper diet can facilitate self-care skills and enhance sense of control over disease.
Encourage the child/adolescent to participate in desired sports or other exercise.	Exercise lowers blood sugar and may decrease insulin needs.
Arrange for child and parent to meet with dietitian.	

Nursing Interventions	Rationales

Teach signs and symptoms of hypoglycemia and hyperglycemia.
1. Hypoglycemia
  • onset rapid (minutes), labile
  • difficulty concentrating, speaking, focusing
  • shaky feeling, dizziness, headache, pallor
  • sweating, tachycardia
  • breath odor normal
  • decreased urine output
  • tremors
  • blood sugar < 60 mg/dL
  • irritable, nervous, weepy
2. Hyperglycemia
  • onset gradual (days)
  • lethargic, dulled sensorium, confused
  • thirst, weakness
  • nausea/vomiting
  • abdominal pain
  • skin flushed, signs of dehydration
  • deep rapid (Kussmaul) respirations
  • fruity acetone breath
  • frequent urination/polyuria
  • blood sugar > 250 mg/dL	

Nursing Interventions	Rationales

Teach child/parent what to do for hypoglycemia:
1. Keep simple carbohydrate on hand.
2. With onset of symptoms, take
  • 120 mL of soft drink (not diet) or orange juice.
  • 2 teaspoons of sugar, honey, or jelly.
  • 4 or 5 hard candies.
3. Repeat twice if needed, but do not over correct.
4. Check blood glucose.
5. Call physician if symptoms do not improve or worsen.
6. Inject glucagon, if instructed.
7. See physician in office or emergency room if needed.	

Teach child/parent what to do for hyperglycemia. 1. Take prescribed dose of insulin. 2. Drink plenty of fluids. 3. Monitor blood glucose. 4. See physician in office or emergency room as directed.	Rarely occurs in children but is possible if dehydrated.
Explain how to manage disease when child is sick: 1. Provide fluids to prevent dehydration. 2. Monitor blood glucose. 3. Call physician for insulin dose adjustment.	
Teach signs/symptoms of impaired circulation.	

▼

DISCHARGE PLANNING/CONTINUITY OF CARE

- Give parent/child emergency phone numbers.
- Encourage participation in Medic-Alert program.
- Provide written materials/guidelines.

- Refer to American Diabetes Association, local chapter.
- Facilitate consults:
  – endocrinology
  – ophthalmology
  – social work
  – visiting nurses
  – dietitian
  – certified diabetes educator

$\mathcal{D}$IAPER RASH (DIAPER DERMATITIS)

Caroline Reich, RN, MS

Diaper rash is a skin irritation in the diaper area (nonallergic, irritant contact dermatitis). This condition is very common in infancy and may be exacerbated by heat, moisture, and sweat retention.

ETIOLOGIES

- Prolonged wetness
- Residual detergents or soaps
- Delay in changing diapers
- Antibiotic usage
- Yeast and bacterial infections

CLINICAL MANIFESTATIONS

- Reddened, inflamed area of convex surfaces (buttocks, medial thighs, mons pubis, and/or scrotum)
- Glistening or glazed appearance with a wrinkled surface

CLINICAL MANIFESTATIONS

None

▼

NURSING DIAGNOSIS: IMPAIRED SKIN INTEGRITY— INFLAMMATION AND RASH

Related To
- Environmental factors (heat, moisture, sweat)
- Chemical substance (irritants)
- Infections

134

Defining Characteristics
See Clinical Manifestations

Patient Outcome
The child will be free of any rashes, inflammation, or excoriation in the diaper region.

Nursing Interventions	Rationales
Obtain a history from the parents of possible contributory factors, onset, appearance, and care practices related to diaper changes and skin care.	
Inspect the infant's entire skin surface, not limiting the exam only to the diaper area.	Underlying skin disorders (such as eczema) may be present.
Show parents how to provide prompt, thorough cleansing of the diaper region with a mild soap and water after each diaper change. Avoid the use of commercially prepared premoistened wipes.	Harsh soaps, chemicals, or overzealous cleansing may damage the epidermis and cause additional inflammation or irritation. This in turn predisposes the infant to greater skin breakdown and secondary infection.
Instruct parent and caregivers to change the infant's diaper after every elimination.	Ammonia (urine) and fecal enzymes that remain on the skin for prolonged periods of time interact to create by-products that cause skin breakdown and maceration.
Demonstrate to parents how to apply a topical layer of steroid cream or ointment to the affected area. Suggest a protective ointment such as Desitin or zinc oxide be used after the most serious inflammation is reduced. Instruct to remove all traces of ointment during cleansing of the diaper area, before reapplication occurs.	Protective ointments such as zinc oxide should not be applied to severely inflamed areas because they tend to exacerbate sweat retention. Zinc oxide tends to stick heavily to skin; it is most easily removed with mineral oil.

Nursing Interventions	Rationales
Obtain physician order for antibiotics if a secondary bacterial or yeast infection exists and instruct parents on use.	Bacterial infections commonly appear as pustulosis. Yeast infections produce a characteristic appearance with erythematous, often papular red patches with a sharply marginated area. Yeast infections usually involve the anterior thighs and abdomen, as well as the diaper area.

▼

NURSING DIAGNOSIS: KNOWLEDGE DEFICIT (CAREGIVER) OF CAUSE OF DIAPER RASH AND TREATMENT NEEDS OF THE AFFECTED AREA

Related To
- Lack of exposure
- Information misinterpretation
- Unfamiliarity with resources

Defining Characteristics
Parents express need for information.
Inaccurate follow-through of instruction.

Patient Outcomes
Parents will verbalize understanding of
- skin care practices to reduce occurrence of diaper rash.
- treatment options available.

Nursing Interventions	Rationales
Assess parents' experience in preventing/treating diaper rash.	
Provide instruction on the various reasons diaper rash occurs, and on good skin care practices such as changing soiled diapers frequently.	Compliance with the treatment regimen is more likely when parents understand the reasons diaper rash may occur and what measures they can undertake to prevent reoccurrences.

Nursing Interventions	Rationales
Instruct to 1. avoid prolonged wetness next to the skin. 2. avoid occlusive diaper coverings such as plastic pants.	Wetness can prevent healing. Occlusive diaper coverings prevent evaporation, thereby increasing maceration from urine breakdown.
Instruct to remove the diaper entirely for extended periods.	This exposes the skin to air, facilitates drying, and reduces unnecessary irritation.
Discuss the advantages and disadvantages to both cloth and disposable diapers in preventing diaper rash. Some infants may be better suited for one type of diaper over another.	It is controversial whether cloth or disposable diapers are better in preventing inflammation and irritation. Disposable diapers with absorbent gelling material increase absorbency and draw wetness away from the skin. A disadvantage to disposables is that, although urine is drawn away from the infant's skin, the urea and ammonia salts that cause skin breakdown are left behind in contact with the infant's skin.
Provide directions on various laundering techniques for cloth diapers: 1. laundering diapers separately 2. using a mild soap (such as Ivory) 3. double rinsing 4. soaking rinsed, soiled diapers in a quaternary ammonium compound (such as Diaperene) or dilute bleach can help disinfect them.	

Nursing Interventions	Rationales
Discuss the benefits and risks of using talcum powder in treating diaper rash.	Diaper rashes involving the skin-folds can be treated by frequent application of unmedicated powder. This will reduce moisture and irritation. Some health care providers believe talcum powder is of questionable benefit because of the risk of aspiration in the infant. Parents need to be taught that talcum powder should be shaken out into the caregiver's hand before application. At no time should powder be shaken around the infant's mouth or nose.
Explain potential use of cornstarch versus powder.	Cornstarch is an absorbable starch that is not readily inhaled; therefore, some health care providers prefer that cornstarch be used if parents insist on using a powder. It is important that parents be taught to remove all traces of wet powder at diaper changes before any additional powder is applied because wet powder also can hold ammonia next to the infant's skin.

▼

DISCHARGE PLANNING/CONTINUITY OF CARE

- Follow up in 2 weeks if no improvement or sooner if condition worsens.
- Refer to dermatologist if needed.

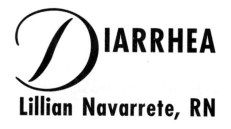

DIARRHEA

Lillian Navarrete, RN

Diarrhea refers to frequent passage of unformed stools and fluid resulting in excessive water and electrolyte loss.

ETIOLOGIES

- Diet
  - idiosyncratic intolerance
  - method of food preparation
  - change in eating schedule/habits
- Level of activity
- Emotional impact—stress/loss of privacy
- Previous gastrointestinal (GI) disease, surgery, or abdominal radiation
- Iatrogenic causes—drugs, GI tests
- Infection—bacterial, viral, parasitic
- Physical abnormality—malabsorption

CLINICAL MANIFESTATIONS

- Green/yellow stool may contain mucus, blood, or pus
- Water, frequent stooling may be explosive
- Abnormal cramps/pain
- Fever
- Irritability
- Lethargy
- Anorexia, vomiting

CLINICAL/DIAGNOSTIC FINDINGS

- Positive cultures if infections
- Positive for ova and parasites

- Stool pH < 6
- Positive reducing substance

▼

NURSING DIAGNOSIS: DIARRHEA

Related To (see Etiologies)

Defining Characteristics
See Clinical Manifestations

Patient Outcome
Child will have normal bowel elimination.

Nursing Interventions	Rationales
Assess history for usual pattern of bowel movements, dietary habits.	An accurate, thorough history will help determine etiology.
Observe or determine description of diarrheal stool, including frequency, odor, and presence of blood or mucus.	
Assess for recent changes in diet, schedule, sleep, exposure to infected individual, medications or psychosocial stress.	New foods may indicate intolerance. Antibiotics frequently cause diarrhea. Changes in school or home situation can stimulate diarrheal stools.
Determine breast-feeding mother's diet and medications.	Mother's diet/medications can be transferred through breast milk and cause side effects.
Determine if others in household have symptoms.	More likely if cause is infectious or due to food spoilage.
Inspect abdomen for distention.	
Auscultate bowel sounds for hyperactivity.	
Palpate for local tenderness, masses, organomegaly.	This is to differentiate from other abdominal disorders. Abdomen should exhibit only generalized tenderness.
Percuss for increased tympany.	
Collect and send stool for ova and parasites and for culture.	This is necessary to identify pathogen.

Nursing Interventions	Rationales
Hematest stool for blood.	
Test stool for pH and reducing substance.	A pH < 6 indicates disaccharide/monosaccharide malabsorption. Positive reducing substance test indicates lactose/glucose malabsorption.
For a child,	
1. Instruct parent to give child clear liquids for 24 hr.	This is to rest the bowel.
2. Advance diet slowly beginning with soft, bland foods.	
For the bottle-fed infant,	
1. Instruct parent to give an oral rehydration solution for first 24 hr, then increase to ½ strength formula for 24 hr.	This is to rest the bowel, while maintaining hydration.
2. If the diarrhea is improving, increase to full strength on third day and slowly reintroduce usual foods beginning with rice cereal.	
For breast-feeding mother,	
1. Encourage mother to avoid foods in her diet that may cause diarrhea in infant (some vegetables, fruits, juices).	
2. Instruct mother to continue nursing but to offer infant water or rehydration solution between feedings for 24 hr.	Breast milk is very easily digested in the infant's intestine and need not be discontinued.
Instruct parent to slowly reintroduce usual diet beginning with bland foods.	
Instruct parent to call or return if diarrhea is not resolving or other symptoms become apparent.	

Nursing Interventions	Rationales
Make sure parent understands need for good hygiene: 1. bottle/formula preparation 2. good handwashing 3. frequent diaper changes and skin care	Poorly washed bottles can be contaminated with spoiled milk or other bacterial growth. Good handwashing diminishes transmissions of contagions. Diarrhea can cause terrible excoriation of skin if not promptly cleaned.

▼

NURSING DIAGNOSIS: FLUID VOLUME DEFICIT

Related To diarrhea

Defining Characteristics
Dry skin, mucous membranes
Poor skin turgor
Decreased urine output
Weight-loss
Low-grade fever
Also for infants: sunken fontanel/eyes, absence of tears when crying

Patient Outcomes
Child's/infant's level of hydration will be normal as evidenced by
• normal weight.
• improved urine output.
• moist skin, mucous membranes.
• level fontanel/eyes.

Nursing Interventions	Rationales
Assess for signs of dehydration.	
Assess vital signs and level of consciousness.	Signs of shock indicate profound dehydration. Child should be hospitalized immediately after stabilization.
Assess for characteristics and duration of diarrhea.	
Determine home care remedies attempted.	

Nursing Interventions	Rationales
Instruct parents to provide adequate fluids, even though foods will be held for 24 hr (see diet instructions under Nursing Diagnosis: Diarrhea).	
Recommend oral rehydration solutions, such as Pedialyte or Litren, over plain water.	Plain water will not improve electrolyte imbalance and rehydration occurs faster with electrolyte solutions. Too much water may cause hypotonic dehydration.
Inform parents of signs of dehydration and the importance of providing fluids.	Dehydration can be life threatening.

▼

DISCHARGE PLANNING/CONTINUITY OF CARE

- Follow up (telephone) in 24 hr.
- Instruct parent to call or return sooner if symptoms worsen, or child refuses fluids or begins vomiting.
- If child/infant is taking antibiotics, consult with prescribing physician—antibiotic may need to be changed or discontinued.
- Refer to pediatrician if diarrhea is prolonged (longer than 4 days), if there is blood in the stool, if infant is under 3 months old, or for dehydration that is not resolving.
- Refer breast-feeding mother to her physician if she is taking antibiotics.

$\mathcal{D}$YSFUNCTIONAL GRIEVING

Kathleen Scharer, RN, MS, CS, FAAN

$\mathbf{D}$ysfunctional grieving refers to an individual's inability to accept and/or mourn a real or perceived loss. It may result in failure to grow, impaired development, or limitation in normal functioning.

ETIOLOGIES

- Actual or perceived object loss
- Thwarted grieving response of a loss
- Absence of anticipatory grieving
- Real or perceived feelings of responsibility for the loss (guilt), often resulting from normal development process of egocentric, magical thinking (9 years or younger)
- Impairment in parental grieving.
- Overwhelming parental grief that interferes with the child's ability to grieve appropriately.
- Lack of support or permission for grieving, including being kept from usual mourning rituals when child is old enough to attend.

CLINICAL MANIFESTATIONS

- Absence of grieving for a significant loss.
- Continual grieving for extended periods interfering with normal development or learning.
- Evidence of clinical depression resulting from the loss.

CLINICAL/DIAGNOSTIC FINDINGS

None necessary

▼

NURSING DIAGNOSIS: DYSFUNCTIONAL GRIEVING

Related To
- Actual or perceived object loss
- Thwarted grieving response to a loss
- Absence of anticipatory grieving
- Chronic fatal illness
- Lack of resolution of previous grieving response
- Loss of significant other
- Loss of personal possession
- Real or perceived feelings of responsibility for the loss (guilt), often resulting from normal development process of egocentric, magical thinking (9 years or younger)
- Feelings of ambivalence toward lost person or object
- Impairment in parental grieving or overwhelming parental grief that interferes the child's ability to grieve appropriately.
- Lack of support or permission for grieving, including being kept from usual mourning rituals when child is old enough to attend
- Multiple other stresses

Defining Characteristics
Idealization of lost object
Developmental regression
Difficulty in expressing loss
Verbal expression of distress over loss
Expression of guilt
Alterations in eating habits, sleep patterns, dream patterns, activity level, libido (for post pubescent adolescents)
Anger
Sadness
Crying
Expression of unresolved issues
Reliving of past experiences
Interference with life functioning
Labile affect
Alteration in concentration and/or pursuit of tasks
Withdrawal from normal activities and relationships
Somatic complaints
Acting out of unresolved issues
Increased aggressive behavior

Patient Outcome
The child no longer demonstrates behavior associated with dysfunctional grieving and resumes previous activities and behavior patterns.

Nursing Interventions	Rationales
Identify behaviors associated with dysfunctional grieving and determine stage of grieving process.	
Identify the perceived or actual lost object and the meaning or value of the object to the patient.	Understanding the value and affective relationship permits appropriate selection of interventions.
Assess family's readiness to permit child's grieving.	If family members are experiencing difficulty in dealing with the loss, they may not be able to support the child's grieving.
Assess any prior experiences with loss and ways used to cope with those losses.	
Identify other current stresses that may interfere with grieving.	If other stressors can be reduced, resolution of dysfunctional grieving may be facilitated.
Assess affective state and evidence of distress.	
Establish a trusting relationship by showing acceptance and listening attentively and empathically.	Trust is the basis of a helping relationship.
Provide opportunities for expression of emotions such as anger and sadness. Utilize play and art media for expression for younger children.	Preadolescent and younger children may be more comfortable expressing their emotions through play and art work than through direct verbalizations. Physical exercise provides a method for sublimating tension and affect. Play allows opportunities for mastery of emotionally difficult experiences.
Encourage family support and permission for grieving, such as reminiscing about lost object or visiting grave.	Family support and modeling may help the child grieve and resolve the loss.
Teach family and older children about normal stages of grief. Provide age-appropriate information for younger children.	

Nursing Interventions	Rationales
Remind child that feelings and wishes cannot harm someone and that the child is not responsible for the loss.	As a result of egocentric magical thinking, child may feel responsible for the loss and needs clarification that feelings themselves do not cause harm.
Teach child and family members that individuals experience some negative as well as positive feelings about others and this is not bad, nor did these feelings cause the loss.	Many people believe you should not speak ill of the dead, but this may impede the child's ability to work through the meaning of the loss if strong ambivalence about the object was present.

▼

DISCHARGE PLANNING/CONTINUITY OF CARE

- Refer child and/or family for therapeutic assistance if necessary. Child or other family members may require psychiatric assistance to resolve grief and deal with any underlying issues.
- Check with school social worker or counselor to see if a support group, such as Rainbows, is available at the child's school.
- Consider a referral to Big Brothers or Big Sisters, if parental grieving has resulted in insufficient adult attention for this child.

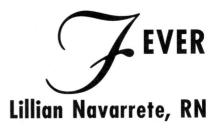

FEVER

Lillian Navarrete, RN

Fever is any abnormal elevation of body temperature.

ETIOLOGIES

- Environmental
- Infectious
- Neurological dysfunction
- Dehydration

CLINICAL MANIFESTATIONS

- Sustained body temperature > 102°F
- Diaphoresis (may not be present in infant)
- Facial flushing
- Warm to touch

CLINICAL/DIAGNOSTIC FINDINGS

Not required for diagnosis

▼

NURSING DIAGNOSIS: HYPERTHERMIA

Related To
- Viral or bacterial infection
- Decreased fluid intake
- Increased fluid output
- Hot environment

Defining Characteristics
Increased temperature
Skin flushing
Diaphoresis
Irritability
Confusion
Hallucinations
Seizures
Tachypnea
Tachycardia
Warm to touch

Patient Outcome
Child's temperature will be < 102°F, rectally.

Nursing Interventions	Rationales
Determine onset and extent of fever.	
Assess for precipitating factors.	Determining and treating the causative factors is essential to controlling fever.
Measure temperature.	
Assess parents' ability to measure temperature at home.	
Assess level of consciousness and for history of seizures.	A sudden, high fever has been associated with seizures.
Assess level of hydration.	Dehydration alone can cause fever.
Explain to parents any other tests necessary to determine etiology, such as throat, urine, or blood cultures.	
Explain etiology once determined, and any treatment prescribed.	
Provide instruction on other measures to control fever:	
1. Offer liquids liberally (tea, colas, Jell-O water, Kool-Aid)	To prevent dehydration.
2. Control environmental temperature; do not overdress.	Overdressing and hot environment will cause diaphoresis and further fluid loss.

Nursing Interventions	Rationales
3. Provide tepid bath, but do not allow child to become chilled.	
4. Medicate with antipyretic.	To control temperature > 102°F.
5. Encourage rest.	

▼

DISCHARGE PLANNING/CONTINUITY OF CARE

- Instruct parents to call or return if fever cannot be controlled, if other signs of infection develop, or if seizures or decrease in level of consciousness occurs.
- Refer for infectious disease or neurological follow-up if fever of unknown origin persists for longer than 4–5 days, or if seizure or other abnormal neurological findings, dehydration, or high fever in infant under 6 months old occurs.

$\mathcal{G}$ASTROESOPHAGEAL REFLUX/PYLORIC STENOSIS

Nedra Skale, RN, MS, CNA

Gastroesophageal reflux (GER) refers to reverse flow of gastric contents up the esophagus. Pyloric stenosis is a thickening of the pyloric muscle that develops in the first month of life.

ETIOLOGIES

GER
- Common in early infancy
- May be due to an immature digestive system
- Overfeeding
- Improper burping

Pyloric Stenosis
- Immature, ineffective function of the pylorus
- Pyloric edema and hypertrophy
- Delayed gastric emptying
- Increased peristalsis

CLINICAL MANIFESTATIONS

Vomiting

CLINICAL/DIAGNOSTIC FINDINGS

Positive
- Upper gastrointestinal (GI) series
- Esophagoscopy
- Biopsy
- Scintiscan

▼

NURSING DIAGNOSIS: ALTERED NUTRITION—LESS THAN BODY REQUIREMENTS

Related To vomiting

Defining Characteristics
Poor/no weight gain
Weight loss

Patient Outcomes
- The infant will consume a well-balanced diet.
- The infant's weight will stabilize and gradually increase.

Nursing Interventions	Rationales
Note the onset, frequency, severity, and timing of the vomiting. Identify precipitating factors such as feeding, coughing, or activity that worsen the vomiting.	Vomiting is the most common symptom of GER in infants. The parent usually will observe that the infant vomits less when held in an upright position. Vomiting in pyloric stenosis is nonbilious. It usually progresses in a few days to the point that every feeding is brought up. This vomiting usually is projectile but also may be regurgitant; it rarely is intermittent. Regurgitation of small amounts of formula soon after each feeding suggests improper feeding techniques, such as inadequate burping or bottle propping.
Note other associated symptoms such as fever, substernal pain, coughing, diarrhea, alterations in mental status, and failure to thrive.	
Identify predisposing conditions, such as a family history in pyloric stenosis or head trauma, hydrocephalus, cerebral palsy, and Down's syndrome in GER.	
Determine the type of formula, manner of preparation, quantity ingested, and feeding position and technique.	
Assess the infant's degree of illness: 1. Take and record baseline vital signs: temperature, pulse, respiratory rate, blood pressure.	

Nursing Interventions	Rationales
2. Plot the infant's weight, height, and head circumference on a grid.	This is to identify an infant with failure to thrive or rapid head growth.
3. Note the presence of irritability, lethargy, seizures, retinal hemorrhages, ataxia, or other focal neurological signs.	Infants who are mildly ill have vomiting associated with feeding but not failure to thrive, and do not have signs of infection or disease. An error in feeding technique or preparation usually is identified as the problem in these cases. Moderately ill infants have failure to thrive, anemia, pneumonia, and signs of infection. Infants with severe illness are dehydrated, have acid-base abnormalities, and may have altered mental status. They are in shock, appear toxic, and may be comatose.
Note the character of the vomitus.	Vomitus of unchanged food and no gastric juice is esophageal. A relaxed cardiac sphincter or rumination will produce small amounts of vomitus with little force. Vomitus with sour milk curds with no green or brown color indicates stomach contents. Vomitus containing greenish-colored fluid indicates the presence of bile and a bowel obstruction.
Explore the possibility of dietary intolerance contributing to the vomiting.	
Obtain a nutritional consult to determine the diet history and required needs for age.	
Instruct the family on the need for diagnostic studies:	
1. Upper GI series to establish if there is GER and to identify abnormalities of the stomach.	If signs and symptoms do not indicate food intolerance, improper feeding, or other illness, further differentiation is necessary.

Nursing Interventions	Rationales
2. pH probe if the upper GI series failed to show GER but the infant still has symptoms.	
3. Scintiscan to establish the frequency of the GER, gastric emptying, and if aspiration is occurring.	
4. Esophagoscopy and biopsy to confirm esophagitis.	

▼

NURSING DIAGNOSIS: HIGH RISK FOR FLUID VOLUME DEFICIT

Risk Factors
- Vomiting
- Inadequate fluid intake

Patient Outcomes
- The infant will maintain adequate intake of fluid and electrolytes.
- The infant's hydration will improve.

Nursing Interventions	Rationales
Assess hydration status: 1. skin/tongue 2. eyes 3. intake and output 4. urine specific gravity 5. color of urine	With dehydration, mucosa (lips, gums) are dry, tongue is dry/furrowed, turgor is decreased, color is pale or flushed, eyeballs are sunken, urine output is greater than intake and is dark, and urine specific gravity is increased.
Record the infant's weight and whether this is an increase or decrease from last visit.	
Assess the infant's temperature.	Fever increases the body's demand for fluid and will worsen an already dehydrated state.
Use tepid sponges and medication as ordered to lower the temperature. Remove excessive clothing.	

Nursing Interventions	Rationales
Encourage parents to continue to feed using proper technique.	
Refer immediately for hospitalization if infant is dehydrated.	Child will require intravenous fluid therapy.

▼

NURSING DIAGNOSIS: HIGH RISK FOR ASPIRATION

Risk Factors
- Excessive or thick secretions/emesis
- Neuromuscular impairment

Patient Outcomes
The patient will
- have optimal movement of air in and out of the lungs.
- not have stasis of air or secretions in the lungs.

Nursing Interventions	Rationales
Assess the child for respiratory distress during and after the vomiting episode.	Frequent vomiting increases risk of aspiration.
Assess for possible defining characteristics of aspiration: 1. episodic aspiration pneumonia 2. abnormal breath sounds—chronic nocturnal wheezing 3. changes in rate and depth of respirations 4. fever 5. cyanosis 6. cough 7. apnea 8. nasal flaring 9. anxiety of restlessness.	
Arrange for chest films if lung sounds are abnormal and pneumonia is suspected.	
Refer infants in distress for hospitalization.	

▼

NURSING DIAGNOSIS: KNOWLEDGE DEFICIT (CAREGIVER)

Related To
- New diagnosis
- Unfamiliarity with necessary treatments

Defining Characteristics

Asks many questions
Verbalized misconceptions
Lack of questions

Patient Outcome

The family will express knowledge of the problem and the solutions proposed by the medical team.

Nursing Interventions	Rationales
Assess the educational needs of the family as they relate to the diagnosis and prescribed treatment.	
Instruct the family on the measures that must be taken with an infant with **GER**:	
1. Change the infant's feeding schedule to small volumes of formula given more frequently to reduce gastric distention (1 oz of thickened feeding for every month of life every 3 hr).	Prevention of gastric distention diminishes the likelihood of food being forced back up into the esophagus.
2. Thicken the formula with cereal (1 tablespoon/oz).	Thickened formula will settle lower in the stomach.
3. Position the infant's body in prone to a 30-degree incline throughout most of the day.	This position allows gravity to keep food in lower portion of stomach.

Nursing Interventions	Rationales
Instruct the family on the natural history of **GER**: 1. Normal infants will grow out of reflux as the lower esophageal sphincter matures and the infant begins to walk. Neurologically impaired infants have an increased risk of serious complications that require surgical treatment. 2. Ninety percent of infants will be well by 15 months of age. 3. Treatment is aimed at controlling symptoms until they spontaneously disappear. 4. Surgery is not necessary in infants unless medical therapy is unsuccessful and the infant's health and life are threatened by continuing complications (apnea, pneumonia).	
Instruct the family on the correct administration of the medications prescribed:	
1. Metoclopramide (Reglan): 0.05– 0.1 mg/kg/dose given 15–20 min prior to feedings.	Increases gastric emptying.
2. Bethanechol (Urocholine): 0.5– 0.75 mg/kg/day given 15–20 min prior to feeding.	Increases peristaltic activity in the stomach and esophagus.
Instruct the family in the care needed for an infant with **pyloric stenosis**:	
1. Once the diagnosis is made by palpation of the olive-sized thickened and enlarged pylorus or by an ultrasound examination or an upper GI series, the infant is admitted to the hospital for intravenous hydration and correction of electrolyte imbalance.	Protracted vomiting results in significant loss of stomach acid, causing hypochloremic alkalosis.

Nursing Interventions	Rationales
2. Surgery always is indicated.	There is no medical treatment for pyloric stenosis.
3. After surgery, feeding is begun in the first 8 hr with small, frequent offerings.	
4. Once full feedings are retained (usually 48 hr after surgery), the infant is discharged.	

▼

DISCHARGE PLANNING/CONTINUITY OF CARE

- For infants with GER, schedule a return visit in 1 week.
- Refer infants with pyloric stenosis to surgeon.
- Arrange Visiting Nurses Association or other home nurse visits to assist parents in learning to care for infant.

$\mathcal{G}$ONORRHEA

Jeffrey Zurlinden, RN, MS

Gonorrhea (GC) is a sexually transmitted disease (STD). It usually causes a localized infection of the urethra, endocervical canal, rectum, or pharynx. The patient may have one site of infection or many sites. The infection is spread by sexual contact with the infected site. Although symptoms abate without treatment, untreated GC may lead to septicemia, pelvic inflammatory disease (PID), and an arthritis-dermatitis syndrome. Unfortunately, it is symptoms of these complications that often cause the infected adolescent to present. Because of late diagnosis, reproductive difficulties may result from scarring. Infection in a young child is suggestive of sexual abuse.

ETIOLOGY

Infection with bacteria *Neisseria gonorrhea*

CLINICAL MANIFESTATIONS

- Asymptomatic
- Thick white-yellow discharge 2–10 days after inoculation at site of infection
- Urinary frequency
- Pain or burning when urinating
- Sore throat
- Mucus or blood in stools
- Change in bowel movements

CLINICAL/DIAGNOSTIC FINDINGS

- Gram-negative intracellular diplococci on smears
- Cultures from infected sites grow *Neisseria gonorrhea.*

▼

NURSING DIAGNOSIS: INFECTION

Related To presence of infectious organisms

Defining Characteristics

Positive culture from urethra, cervix, throat, or rectum
Gram-negative intracellular diplococci on smear
History of sexual contact with an infected person

Patient Outcomes

Child/adolescent will exhibit no signs of infection, as evidenced by resolution of discharge or negative test-of-cure culture.

Nursing Interventions	Rationales
Check local and state regulations to determine if STDs in minors are reportable to the health department.	
Determine date of last sexual contact, number of sexual partners, and description of recent sexual activities.	Provides information regarding behaviors that increase risk of STDs.
Obtain cultures from all sites of possible infection.	Women frequently self-inoculate their rectums with GC from urethral or endocervical discharges. Because cold culture medium is bacteriocidal, warm Thayer Martin culture plates to room temperature before inoculation. Store inoculated plates in CO_2 enriched environment to prevent death of *Neisseria gonorrhea* from room air O_2 concentrations.
Obtain smears from discharges.	
Obtain history of previous STDs.	Although GC can be treated effectively with antibiotics, the cure will not prevent future recurrences of the disease.

Nursing Interventions	Rationales
Assess	
1. urethral and/or cervical discharge.	Frequently asymptomatic. If symptomatic, thick yellow-white discharge occurs 2–10 days after infection.
2. urinary frequency.	
3. pain or burning when urinating.	
4. rectal discharge.	Frequently asymptomatic. If symptomatic, thick yellow-white discharge occurs 2–10 days after infection.
5. mucus or blood in stools.	
6. change in bowel movements.	
7. sore throat.	Pharyngeal GC usually is asymptomatic.
Screen for other STDs, hepatitis B, and human immunodeficiency virus (HIV).	Patients with one STD are at higher risk for a concomitant STD. Thirty to 40% of women with GC also are infected with chlamydia and may require treatment with additional antibiotics.
In women, obtain menstrual history, including date of last period.	It can be difficult to get cultures during menstruation; results are less accurate (increased number of false negatives), especially with tampon use.
Determine method of and compliance with birth control.	Contracting STDs suggests no use/improper use of condoms, which also increases the risk for pregnancy. Nurse should use this opportunity for health screening/education.
Check local/state regulations to determine if minors can receive abortion or birth control counseling without parental notification or consent.	

Nursing Interventions	Rationales
Perform pregnancy test.	Necessary for early detection of pregnancy. Young women can become pregnant before menarche. Some drugs have teratogenic effect.
Check local/state regulations to determine if minors can receive treatment for STDs without parenteral notification or consent.	
Administer antibiotics as ordered.	Treatment for GC frequently changes in response to the introduction of new antibiotics and new resistant strains of GC. Follow the current guidelines from the Centers for Disease Control (CDC) or local Health Department.
Observe for possible anaphylactic reaction to intramuscular (IM) antibiotics given during clinic visit.	
Dispense condoms.	Latex condoms are the most effective means of preventing spread of disease during sexual contact.
Instruct patient to inform all recent sexual partners of possible exposure to GC and need for treatment.	Untreated asymptomatic sexual partners are common source of reinfection
Determine if sexual contact was consensual. Refer to social services if sexual abuse is suspected.	

▼

NURSING DIAGNOSIS: KNOWLEDGE DEFICIT

Related To new diagnosis

Defining Characteristics
Asks many questions
Asks few questions
History of repeated infections
Patient is unable to state the causes, treatment, and prevention of GC

Patient Outcomes

Patient will state
- medication schedule.
- medication side effects.
- date of return visit for test of cure.
- how to use condoms to prevent future infections.

Nursing Interventions	Rationales
Assess patient's present level of understanding.	Misconceptions can increase anxiety/fear and foster spread of STD.
Instruct patient about medication schedule and side effects of antibiotics used to treat GC.	Treatment for GC frequently changes in response to the introduction of new antibiotics and new resistant strains of GC. Follow the current guidelines from the CDC or local Health Department.
Instruct patient to refrain from vaginal, rectal, and pharyngeal sexual intercourse until partners are treated and results are reported from test-of-cure culture.	
Instruct patient on mode of transmission: local inoculation of bacteria from partner's penis to patient's throat, vagina, or rectum.	
Instruct patient to use latex condoms or use other nonintercourse sexual methods to prevent future infections.	Latex condoms are an effective barrier against GC.
Inform patient of the possible consequences of untreated GC.	PID, ectopic pregnancy, or difficulty conceiving as a result of scarred fallopian tubes are common complications.

▼

NURSING DIAGNOSIS: INEFFECTIVE MANAGEMENT OF THERAPEUTIC REGIMEN

Related To
- Unwillingness to comply with treatment, prevention, or informing sexual partners
- Complexity of treatment regimen

Defining Characteristics

Persistent infection not caused by antibiotic-resistant strains
Missed return visit for test of cure
Incorrect pill count at return visit
Inadequate blood level of antibiotic

Patient Outcomes

Patient will
- complete course of treatment.
- notify sexual partners.
- return for test-of-cure culture.
- use condoms to prevent infection.

Nursing Interventions	Rationales
Compare actual effect and expected therapeutic effect.	
Plot patient's pattern of returning for tests of cure or follow-up visits.	
Determine social support system and presence of significant others.	Interpersonal influence can impact on compliance with treatment regimen.
Assess patient's and significant other's beliefs about current illness and treatment plan.	How one views perceived susceptibility, severity, and threat of disease impacts on health behavior.
Assess quality of relationship between patient and health care workers and health care facility.	
Role play to practice informing sexual partners of possible exposure to GC.	This gives patient opportunity to rehearse situation and allows nurse to provide feedback.
Suggest IM medications or short-term therapy, if patient has a history of not taking oral medication.	IM medication eliminates the patient's need to participate in treatment.
Role play to practice new behaviors in situations leading to reinfection (such as saying "no" or using condoms).	
Develop a positive relationship with the patient that encourages participation with treatment decisions.	The nurse-patient relationship is based on recognition of patient's right to self-determination and capacity for self-management, with focus on decision making and goal attainment.

Nursing Interventions	Rationales
Determine with the patient the plan of treatment he/she is most likely to complete.	Involving the patient in planning the regimen improves compliance.

▼

NURSING DIAGNOSIS: ALTERED SEXUALITY PATTERNS

Related To
- Imposed restrictions
- Fear
- Risk of contagion

Defining Characteristics
Patient or significant other expresses concern about the effects GC and treatment have on their expressions of physical intimacy.

Patient Outcome
Patient will state ways of expressing physical intimacy during treatment.

Nursing Interventions	Rationales
Determine patient's or significant other's concerns.	STD diagnosis may provoke feelings of guilt, shame, the need for punishment, or other anxiety-provoking thoughts unique to the patient.
Determine if patient's or significant other's concerns also are related to fears about acquired immunodeficiency syndrome (AIDS).	An STD diagnosis may provoke fear of AIDS that alters sexual behavior.
Assess perception of meaning of GC infection.	This provides opportunity to correct misconceptions.
Elicit patient's feeling about limits on sexual behavior.	
Interview patient in a quiet, private, distraction-free environment.	Adolescents are hesitant to discuss personal sexual matters. The proper setting may facilitate discussion.
Explore ways to express physical intimacy that do not lead to reinfection.	Barrier contraception with latex condoms is effective.

▼

DISCHARGE PLANNING/CONTINUITY OF CARE

- Arrange gynecology consult.
- Schedule patient to return to the clinic to obtain culture to demonstrate test of cure. (Antibiotic-resistant strains cause treatment failures that can be detected only by test of cure culture.)
- Instruct patient to return for routine screening if high-risk sexual behavior continues.
- Instruct patient to report persistence or recurrence of symptoms.
- Refer
  – for HIV counseling and testing
  – to family planning clinic
  – to support group

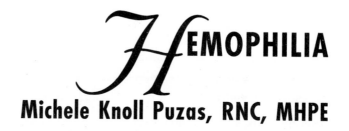

HEMOPHILIA

Michele Knoll Puzas, RNC, MHPE

Hemophilia is an inherited disorder that results in inadequate blood levels of coagulation factors. A deficiency in coagulation factors causes prolonged and inappropriate bleeding.

ETIOLOGY

X-linked recessive inheritance

CLINICAL MANIFESTATIONS

- Easy bruising
- Prolonged bleeding
- Greater than usual blood loss during dental procedures
- Epistaxis
- Hemarthrosis
- Internal hemorrhage
- Hematuria

CLINICAL/DIAGNOSTIC FINDINGS

- Hemophilia A—deficiency or absence of antihemophilia factor VIII
- Hemophilia B (Christmas disease)—deficiency or absence of factor IX

▼

NURSING DIAGNOSIS: HIGH RISK FOR INJURY

Risk Factors
- Inadequate or absent clotting factors
- Altered mobility
- Developmental level

Patient Outcomes

- The child will be protected from injury as evidenced by adherence to preventive practices.
- Bleeding episodes will be controlled.

Nursing Interventions	Rationales
Determine type of hemophilia, if known.	
Assess for obvious bleeding.	
Apply pressure, ice, or topical hemostatic agent.	This is to limit blood loss.
Refer immediately to hospital emergency room for severe or uncontrolled bleeding, or if internal hemorrhage or head injury is suspected.	Significant blood loss is life threatening.
Assess for joint swelling, limitation of movement, and pain. Obtain x-rays.	These findings may indicate bleeding/hemarthrosis.
If joint bleeding is suspected, immobilize joint in position of slight flexion. Elevate affected part and apply ice.	Extreme positioning may increase bleeding and development of contractures.
Determine bleeding time, partial thromboplastin time, and hematocrit.	Prolonged partial thromboplastin time or bleeding time indicate decreased factor level.
Administer antihemophiliac factor. Factor replacements include 1. fresh frozen plasma 2. cryoprecipitates 3. lyophilized concentrates	Bleeding will not be controlled without factor replacement.
Instruct parents on wound/joint care and factor administration at home.	Child and parent must know how to manage care at home; hemophilia is a lifelong condition.

Nursing Interventions	Rationales
Determine prevention measures the child and family can employ to reduce risk of injury. Encourage 1. avoiding contact sports 2. use of acetominophen instead of aspirin for pain or fever 3. gentle oral hygiene 4. avoiding rectal temperature measurement 5. administering prescribed factor.	This maintains adequate blood levels to decrease risk of significant bleeding.

▼

NURSING DIAGNOSIS: PAIN

Related To
- Bleeding into joⁱ
- Trauma

Defining Characteristics
Moaning
Crying
Irritability
Verbal expression of pain

Patient Outcome
The child will verbalize adequate pain control.

Nursing Interventions	Rationales
Assess pain 1. site 2. onset 3. severity 4. duration 5. cause 6. relief factors	Assessment of pain provides guidance for treatment.
Assess mobility, but avoid excessive manipulation.	Diminished mobility may indicate bleeding into the joint; excessive manipulation will increase bleeding and pain.
Immobilize affected joint and apply ice.	Ice will diminish pain sensation as well as swelling.

Nursing Interventions	Rationales
Treat wound/bruise pain with acetaminophen and ice.	
Send home with instructions for pain control.	
1. Joint pain • Immobilize during acute phase. • Continue ice applications. • Administer acetaminophen, or codeine for severe pain.	
• Provide diversional activities.	Can be effective in reducing perception of pain.
• Begin passive range of motion after pain has diminished.	Maintains muscle strength and joint function. Repeated episodes of hemarthrosis are extremely destructive to bone structure and joint function.
2. Bruise/wound pain • Administer acetaminophen. • Apply cold packs. (Severe or increasing pain indicates a need to return to health care provider.)	

▼

NURSING DIAGNOSIS: HIGH RISK FOR INEFFECTIVE COPING (CHILD/PARENTS)

Risk Factors
• Life-threatening condition
• Unsatisfactory support system
• Unrealistic perceptions
• Anxiety/fear

Patient Outcomes
Child/family will
• verbalize acceptance of hemophilia.
• seek out appropriate support resources.

Nursing Interventions	Rationales
Assess child/family's past/current coping abilities, noting strengths, problems, and resources.	Individuals with unsuccessful coping in past may need additional resources.
Encourage questions and verbalization of fears/concerns.	Misconceptions can increase anxiety and damage self-concept.
Acknowledge the normalcy of concerns about living with hemophilia.	
Explore attitudes about needed life-style changes.	This is a lifelong condition, and adherence to preventive measures will be lifesaving. However, children have difficulty being different from their peers.
For older child, encourage participation in self-help groups as available.	Support groups provide a realistic picture of the condition and guidance with potential/actual problems.
Discuss the use of factor preparations and blood transfusions. Inform child and family of reduced risk for human immunodeficiency virus (HIV) or hepatitis.	Since 1986, donated blood has been screened for HIV and hepatitis.
Discuss the importance of HIV testing for the child who received blood or factor products prior to 1986.	Early detection of positive HIV status allows for early initiation of treatment.

▼

DISCHARGE PLANNING/CONTINUITY OF CARE

- Teach parent/child
  - about disease and treatment
  - safety measures
  - home administration of factor preparation
  - emergency techniques and when to get help
- Arrange home intravenous therapy if needed.
- Provide information on support groups.
- Refer for physical therapy.
- Arrange genetic counseling when needed.
- Determine frequency of medical/dental follow-up based on individual child/family needs.
- Facilitate obtaining Medic-Alert identification.

$\mathcal{H}$ERNIA, INGUINAL

Nedra Skale, RN, MS, CNA

An inguinal hernia is a protrusion of an abdominal viscus into a peritoneal sac (processus vaginalis) in the inguinal canal. The content of the sac is usually intestine but also may be ovary, bladder, omentum, or fallopian tube. It is a common defect occurring six times more frequently in males than females. The incidence also is increased in premature infants and children with Ehler-Danlos syndrome, exstrophy of the bladder, or a ventriculoperitoneal shunt.

ETIOLOGY

Congenital defect—failure of the processus vaginalis to close during the last month of fetal life

CLINICAL MANIFESTATIONS

- Observable bulge in the groin
- Palpable bulge along the inguinal canal, scrotum, labia, or anterior thigh

CLINICAL/DIAGNOSTIC FINDINGS

None required

▼

NURSING DIAGNOSIS: PAIN
Related To
- Inflammed tissue
- Incarcerated bowel
- Obstruction of bowel

Defining Characteristics

Facial mask of pain
Crying, moaning
Guarded position
Increased pulse, blood pressure, and respirations
Dilated pupils
Restlessness
Hard, tender, fixed mass in the groin
Does not want to be left alone

Patient Outcomes

- The child's pain will be eliminated.
- The hernia will be reduced.

Nursing Interventions	Rationales
Obtain the child's medical history. Was the child premature? Has there been trauma to the area of the mass?	There is an increased incidence with premature infants.
Obtain the history of the inguinal mass. When was it first noticed? On which side was it noticed? Does activity or crying make the mass larger? Is the child irritable at times for an unknown reason?	Nearly half of all inguinal hernias are noted in the first year of life, most in the first 6 months. Typically, the hernia appears when the child cries or strains but disappears when he/she relaxes. If the hernia has been present for a long time, it may remain out constantly.
Assess for and document clinical evidence that is characteristic of an incarcerated hernia: 1. sudden onset 2. severe pain 3. a hard, tender, fixed mass in the groin 4. symptoms of intestinal obstruction (vomiting and distention) 5. no prior history of a hernia	An inguinal hernia is not painful unless incarcerated.

Nursing Interventions	Rationales
If there is a suggestion that the hernia is incarcerated, notify the physician immediately.	
1. Inform parents of need to attempt reduction of hernia.	Reduction of an incarcerated hernia always should be attempted because operating on an incarcerated hernia carries an increased risk of complications, primarily wound infections, and an increased risk of recurrence.
2. Explain to parents techniques to reduce hernia:	
• Apply steady pressure to mass.	Almost all incarcerated hernias can be reduced with sedation and firm steady pressure applied to the mass for several minutes. As the edema is squeezed out of the bowel wall, it becomes smaller and reducible.
• Position child in head-down position.	The head-down position allows gravity to help with the reduction.
• Prepare parents/child to accept that, if the hernia cannot be reduced, surgery is indicated immediately.	
After reduction, prepare the child for admission to the hospital for observation.	This is to determine that no damage was done to the intestines or testes and to observe for recurrent incarcerations.

▼

NURSING DIAGNOSIS: FEAR

Related To
• Abnormal finding
• Child's pain
• Proposed treatment
• Lack of information

Defining Characteristics

Apprehension regarding proposed surgery
Jittery
Panicked
Frightened
Crying

Patient Outcomes

The child and/or family verbalize
• fears related to surgery and a realistic perception of the danger.
• expectations of the postoperative period.

Nursing Interventions	Rationales
Assess the educational needs of the child and/or family as related to the treatment recommended.	An inguinal hernia will not spontaneously resolve.
Inform the family of what an inguinal hernia is and the cause.	Improved understanding will help alleviate fear.
Reinforce the need for surgical repair of the inguinal hernia.	All inguinal hernias should be repaired promptly unless there are other medical conditions that make the risk of surgery prohibitive. Spontaneous disappearance of the hernia does *not* occur. The risk of incarceration is greater in the small, premature baby. Premature infants should be operated on before they go home from the hospital; normal newborns should be operated on soon after discharge. With the advent of safer anesthesia techniques (spinal anesthesia) for pediatric patients there is no advantage to waiting to repair an inguinal hernia until the child gets older.
Teach the family the specifics of the surgery and the expected postoperative recovery.	This is usually an outpatient procedure; parents need to understand pre- and postoperative requirements.

Nursing Interventions	Rationales
Reinstruct the family on what they should look for and do at home should incarceration occur prior to surgical repair: 1. Place child's head down with buttocks on pillow. 2. Gently massage the inguinal mass with the fingertips, trying to push it up toward the child's head. 3. If massage does not decrease the mass, hold the mass between the fingers and gently squeeze, as for a tube of toothpaste, toward the head. 4. If this still does not reduce the hernia, bring the child to the emergency room immediately.	

▼

DISCHARGE PLANNING/CONTINUITY OF CARE

- Initiate referral to pediatric surgeon.
- Initial follow-up (postoperative) will be with surgeon.
- Follow-up by primary care provider as needed.

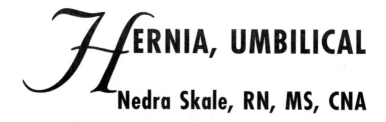

HERNIA, UMBILICAL

Nedra Skale, RN, MS, CNA

An umbilical hernia is the herniation of intestine or omentum through a fascial defect in the umbilicus. Failure of the umbilical ring to contract as the intestines return to the celomic cavity leaves a fascial defect at the exit of the umbilical cord. It is a common defect, occurring 5–10 times more frequently in blacks than whites. The incidence also is increased in children with Beckwith's syndrome, trisomy 13 or 18, and Hurler's syndrome.

ETIOLOGY

Congenital

CLINICAL MANIFESTATIONS

Protruding umbilicus

CLINICAL/DIAGNOSTIC FINDINGS

None

▼

NURSING DIAGNOSIS: BODY IMAGE DISTURBANCE

Related To
- Abnormal physical appearance
- Lack of information

Defining Characteristics
Refusal to touch or look at the body part
Withdrawal from social contacts

Self-destructive behavior
Unwillingness to discuss the defect

Patient Outcomes
- The child will
    - participate in school and social activities.
    - not demonstrate self-destructive behavior.
- The child/family will recognize the value of the treatment recommended.

Nursing Interventions	Rationales
Obtain the natural history of umbilical hernia (is it getting smaller, staying the same or enlarging?).	Because 95% of umbilical hernias disappear by age 5, operative repair seldom is necessary.
Assess the history for evidence of incarceration.	Children who have pain or incarceration and those whose defect is large require operative repair. Spontaneous closure of a defect 2 cm or greater is unlikely. Also, because of the life-threatening risk of complications during pregnancy, females should have operative closure before they reach childbearing age.
Assess the educational needs of the child and family as they relate to the treatment recommended.	
Because the sight of the hernia usually is disconcerting to the parents, provide reassurance regarding the innocuous nature of the defect.	
Instruct the family that taping or strapping the hernia is of no value in expediting the closure and may cause skin irritation.	Misconceptions regarding optimal treatment are common.
Assess the child's reaction to having and looking at the defect.	The perception of change is strongly influenced by child's age and developmental level. School-age children, especially, are conscious of their body and react to being different from classmates. Classmates also may make fun of a child with a hernia.

Nursing Interventions	Rationales
Acknowledge the normalcy of the child's response.	
When appropriate, emphasize the temporary nature of the hernia.	Most close by age 5.
Assist child/parent to utilize prior coping techniques.	
If the child is having great difficulty coping with the hernia, suggest talking to surgeon regarding possibility of surgery.	

▼

DISCHARGE PLANNING/CONTINUITY OF CARE

- Instruct the family to seek immediate medical attention if the child complains of severe pain at the site of the defect. (Strangulation or incarceration of herniated bowel is rare but requires immediate surgical intervention if it cannot be reduced with sedation and gentle manipulation.)
- Follow up at subsequent routine visits.

$\mathcal{H}$ERPES

Jeffrey Zurlinden, RN, MS

Herpes is one of the most common sexually transmitted diseases (STDs). It is a chronic viral infection that results in periodic outbreaks of blisters. The blisters shed virus that may cause new infections at the site of contact with traumatized skin or mucous membranes. The disease most often is seen in sexually active adolescents, as well as adults. Because herpes can cause serious, life-threatening infections in newborns, pregnant women require cesarean section. Infection in a child may indicate sexual abuse.

ETIOLOGY

Infection with herpes simplex virus (HSV) types I and II

CLINICAL MANIFESTATIONS

Prodromal symptoms
- Fatigue
- Malaise
- Headache
- Enlarged or tender lymph nodes

Followed by
- Clusters of itching, burning, painful vesicles that coalesce and then erode

CLINICAL/DIAGNOSTIC FINDINGS

Positive cultures (HSV)

▼

NURSING DIAGNOSIS: INFECTION

Related To presence of infectious organisms

Defining Characteristics
Painful vesicles
Culture positive for HSV

Patient Outcomes
- Patient's vesicles will heal.
- No additional sites of infection will develop.

Nursing Interventions	Rationales
Check local and state regulations to determine if STDs in minors are reportable to the health department.	
Determine date of last sexual contact, number of sexual partners, and description of recent sexual activities.	This provides information regarding behaviors that increase risk of STD.
Obtain cultures (may be unnecessary)	
Obtain history of previous STDs.	
Inspect the perineum, vagina, penis, rectum, and mouth for vesicles.	
Ask about constitutional symptoms, such as fatigue, headache, malaise, and muscle ache, and localized symptoms, such as pain, itching, burning, paresthesia, and tender or swollen regional lymph nodes.	This is to detect associated complications that may require treatment.
Screen for other STDs, hepatitis B, and human immunodeficiency virus (HIV).	Patients with one STD are at higher risk for a concomitant STD.
For women, obtain menstrual history, including date of last period.	It can be difficult to get cultures during menstruation; results are less accurate (more false negatives), especially with tampon use.
Determine method of and compliance with birth control.	Contracting STDs suggests no use/improper use of condoms. Adolescent may be at higher risk for pregnancy. Nurse should use this opportunity for health screening/education.

Nursing Interventions	Rationales
Check local and state regulations to determine if minors can receive abortion or birth control counseling without parental notification or consent.	
Perform pregnancy test.	This is necessary for early detection of pregnancy. Young women can become pregnant before menarche. Some drugs have teratogenic effect. If the virus is active during a pregnancy, the baby can be at risk.
Check local and state regulations to determine if minors can receive treatment for STDs without parental notification or consent.	
Administer acyclovir (Zovirax) as ordered, usually 200 mg five times daily for 10 days for initial outbreak. Patient with frequent outbreaks may receive chronic suppressive therapy with 200 mg three times daily.	
For subsequent outbreaks, instruct patient to start medication at the time of the first sensation of tingling.	Medication is most effective if started early.
Dispense condoms.	Because virus continues to shed through healed lesions, condoms are necessary even after vesicles heal.
Instruct patient to wash hands on waking and after using the bathroom.	Frequent handwashing during outbreaks prevents spreading virus to new sites.
Instruct patient to wash genital lesions with mild soap and dry with a blow dryer.	
Determine if sexual contact was consensual. Refer to social services if suspected sexual abuse.	

▼

NURSING DIAGNOSIS: KNOWLEDGE DEFICIT

Related To new diagnosis

Defining Characteristics
Asks many questions
Asks few questions
Unable to state the causes, treatment, and ways to prevent spreading HSV

Patient Outcomes
Patient will state
- medication schedule and side effects.
- how to use condoms to prevent new site of infection.
- how virus is transmitted and reactivated.
- the effects of stress on outbreaks.

Nursing Interventions	Rationales
Assess patient's present level of understanding.	Misconceptions can increase anxiety/fear and foster spread of STD.
Instruct about medication schedule and side effects of acyclovir.	Oral medications may be prescribed for 5 days to 6 months, depending whether this is an initial, recurrent, or chronic infection.
Instruct to refrain from sexual intercourse involving the infected part of the body during outbreaks, starting at the time of the first sensation of tingling.	
Instruct on mode of transmission: local inoculation of virus from the vesicles to the patient's or partner's traumatized skin or mucous membranes.	During outbreaks, the patient also may inoculate virus to new sites of his/her body—for example, by scratching vesicles and then rubbing his/her eyes without first washing hands.
Instruct patient to use latex condoms or use other nonintercourse sexual methods to prevent future infections.	Latex condoms reduce the risk of spreading the virus. Because the virus may be shed for many months through healed skin, condoms are necessary even after the vesicles heal.

Nursing Interventions	Rationales
Inform of the possible consequences of untreated HSV during pregnancy: infection of the newborn as he/she passes through the birth canal.	HSV may cause serious, life-threatening infections in newborns.
Inform patient that herpes is a chronic infection with periods of exacerbation and remission.	
Inform patient that stress may precipitate outbreaks.	Stress may be emotional stress or physical stress, such as other infections, menses, or prolonged exposure to the sun or heat.

▼

NURSING DIAGNOSIS: INEFFECTIVE MANAGEMENT OF THERAPEUTIC REGIMEN

Related To
- Unwillingness to comply with treatment, prevention, or informing sexual partners
- Complexity of treatment regimen

Defining Characteristics
Frequent outbreaks
Incorrect pill count at return visit

Patient Outcomes
Patient will
- complete course of treatment.
- notify sexual partners.
- use condoms to prevent new sites of infection.

Nursing Interventions	Rationales
Compare actual effect and expected therapeutic effect.	
Determine social support systems and presence of significant others.	Interpersonal influence can impact on compliance with treatment regimen.
Assess beliefs about current illness and treatment plan.	How one perceives susceptibility, severity, and threat of disease impacts on health behaviors.

Nursing Interventions	Rationales
Assess quality of relationship between patient and health care workers and health care facility.	
Role play to practice informing sexual partners of HSV infection.	This gives patient an opportunity to rehearse situations and allows nurse to provide feedback.
Develop a positive relationship with the patient that encourages participation in treatment decisions.	The nurse-patient relationship is based on recognition of patient's right to self-determination and capacity for self-management, with focus on decision making and goal attainment.
Determine with the patient the plan of treatment he/she is most likely to complete.	Involving the patient in planning the regimen improves compliance.

▼

NURSING DIAGNOSIS: ALTERED SEXUALITY PATTERNS

Related To
- Imposed restrictions
- Fear
- Risk of contagion

Defining Characteristics
Patient or significant other expresses concern about the effects herpes has on the expressions of physical intimacy

Patient Outcome
Patient will state ways of expressing physical intimacy during a herpes outbreak.

Nursing Interventions	Rationales
Determine patient's or significant other's concerns.	STD diagnosis may provoke feelings of guilt, shame, the need for punishment, or other anxiety-provoking thoughts unique to patient.
Determine if concerns also are related to fears about acquired immunodeficiency syndrome (AIDS).	An STD diagnosis may provoke fear of AIDS that alters sexual behavior.

Nursing Interventions	Rationales
Assess perception of meaning of herpes infection.	This provides opportunity to correct misconceptions.
Explore ways to express physical intimacy during outbreaks excluding vaginal, rectal, and pharyngeal intercourse.	Restrictions on sexual activity should not deprive the couple of other activities that convey the message that they are loved and desired.
Elicit patient's feelings about limits on sexual behavior.	

▼

DISCHARGE PLANNING/CONTINUITY OF CARE

- Arrange gynecology consult.
- Instruct patient to report persistence or recurrent of symptoms.
- Refer
    - for counseling and testing
    - to family planning clinic
    - for stress management
    - to support group
- Instruct patient, if she becomes pregnant, to notify physician of history of herpes.

IDIOPATHIC THROMBOCYTOPENIC PURPURA

Sandra N. Roberts, RN, MSN

Idiopathic thrombocytopenic purpura (ITP) is an acquired blood disorder that is characterized by increased destruction of circulating platelets. The pathophysiology includes platelets becoming coated with autoplatelet antibody; as a result, they are recognized as foreign material and destroyed by the spleen.

ETIOLOGY

Unknown

CLINICAL MANIFESTATIONS

- Easy bruising with generalized petechiae
- Ecchymosis
- Epistasis
- Bleeding from other mucous membranes
- Positive history of a recent febrile illness

CLINICAL/DIAGNOSTIC FINDINGS

- Platelet count < 20,000–30,000 mm^3/dL
- Increased bleeding time
- Heme-positive urine/stool

▼

NURSING DIAGNOSIS: HIGH RISK FOR INJURY (EASY BRUISING AND BLEEDING)

Risk Factor
- Autoimmune destruction of platelets

Patient Outcomes
- The child will have minimal bruising/bleeding.
- The child's platelet count will be normal or elevated.

Nursing Interventions	Rationales
Assess skin for appearance of petechiae and ecchymosis.	Random petechiae and ecchymosis may occur over entire body.
Observe for bleeding from mucous membranes.	
Assess vital signs for changes: 1. tachycardia 2. hypotension	Significant hemodynamic changes denote extensive blood loss.
Monitor laboratory values (i.e., complete blood count, platelets.	ITP is characterized by reduced platelet count (< 20,000–30,000 mm^3/dL), higher than normal levels of megakaryocytes (parent cell of platelet) on bone marrow aspiration, and prolonged bleeding time.
Perform dipstick test of urine, guaiac or Hematest of stools.	These tests determine presence of blood, which guides subsequent treatment.
Administer one of the possible treatment drugs for ITP as ordered: steroids, high-dose gammaglobulin.	These substances are used to elevate the platelet count.
Assure that invasive procedures (i.e., intramuscular injections or venipunctures) are performed by an experienced skilled clinician.	Protects child from therapeutically induced trauma, limits new petechiae and areas of ecchymosis, and prevents prolonged bleeding.

Nursing Interventions	Rationales
Inform child/parents that severe bleeding and/or dangerously low platelet counts will necessitate hospitalization with the possibility of transfusion therapy or splenectomy.	Antiplatelet antibodies are produced by the spleen.

▼

NURSING DIAGNOSIS: FEAR (FAMILY AND INDIVIDUAL)

Related To concern that child may have a life-threatening illness

Defining Characteristics

Parents frightened to discover their child covered with bruises
Fearful of child "bleeding to death" if bleeding from mucous membranes
Verbalized lack of understanding of disease
Frequent questions and concerns
Difficult for parents to accept that "no treatment" may be the acceptable treatment

Patient Outcomes

The child/family will verbalize
- an understanding of disorder and treatment.
- decreased fear regarding diagnosis.

Nursing Interventions	Rationales
Assess parents'/child's level of fear.	This provides baseline for care planning.
Assess parents'/child's knowledge level regarding diagnosis, treatment and prognosis of ITP.	This provides opportunity to correct misconception.
Inform/reassure parents/child about progress of the disease and its treatment.	The majority of patients recover spontaneously in 6–12 months. Fear is reduced when the reality of the condition is confronted.
Assist family to identify and utilize effective coping mechanisms.	Increases sense of control, which can reduce sense of fear/powerlessness.

Nursing Interventions	Rationales
Determine child/parent level of motivation to maintain home treatment program.	In order for regimen to be effective, child/parent must be involved. Learning only takes place when readiness and interest are demonstrated.
Instruct parent/child to avoid injury:	Knowledge of high-risk behaviors enhances compliance with possible treatment.
1. Avoid rough, injury-prone activities such as contact sports, climbing trees, and riding motorcycles. 2. Move furniture with sharp edges and throw rugs for duration of illness. 3. Normal toppling and frequent falls of a toddler usually are not dangerous. 4. Use soft toothbrush to brush teeth. 5. Monitor child when he/she is using scissors or other sharp objects. 6. Caution child not to blow nose forcefully and not to sneeze with mouth closed. 7. Avoid constipation; ensure adequate fluids, fiber, and exercise. Avoid enemas. 8. Avoid rectal temperatures.	
9. Caution parents to avoid giving their child aspirin or aspirin-containing products.	These inhibit platelet aggregation.
Instruct parents to assess child for bruising and bleeding.	Child may not be aware of bruises, or may be unable to assess entire body.

Nursing Interventions	Rationales
Instruct parents on emergency procedure for increased bleeding or serious injury: 1. Notify health center immediately. 2. Observe for symptoms of central nervous system bleeding (i.e., headaches, diplopia, projectile vomiting, lethargy, sensorium changes).	Early assessment and prompt treatment may reduce potential complications.

▼

DISCHARGE PLANNING/CONTINUITY OF CARE

- Instruct parents on signs and symptoms of hemorrhage (pale diaphoretic skin, decreased urine output, or confusion) indicating need for emergent care.
- Emphasize the need for close follow-up by physician:
  – Platelet counts will be measured every 1–2 weeks.
- Initiate referrals with public health nurse or other agency that can assist in overall management.

$\mathcal{I}$MPETIGO

Ruth Novitt Schumacher, RN, MSN

Impetigo is an inflammatory skin disease marked by isolated pustules that become crusty and rupture.

ETIOLOGIES

Infection with
- Group A streptococci
- *Staphylococcus aureus*
- A combination of both

CLINICAL MANIFESTATIONS

- Presence of skin lesions from macules to draining vesicles
- Pruritis

CLINICAL/DIAGNOSTIC FINDINGS

Positive cultures of exudate

▼

NURSING DIAGNOSIS: IMPAIRED SKIN INTEGRITY

Related To overgrowth of bacterial flora on skin

Defining Characteristics
Red macules
Vesicles
Honey-colored exudate
Pruritis

Patient Outcome
Child's skin will heal without evidence of scarring.

Nursing Interventions	Rationales
Assess for history of exposure and for history of minor skin trauma such as scratches or insect bites.	A break in skin integrity increases risk of infection.
Assess skin from head to toe, with the child as completely undressed as possible.	This is necessary to obtain a thorough evaluation of extent of involvement.
Assess lesions for location and type.	Minor infection may require only cleansing and topical medication.
Instruct the parents on cleansing skin with antiseptic soap and applying bacteriocidal ointment. Use a disposable applicator (cotton swab) so lesions are not touched directly.	An understanding of the importance of good technique can improve compliance.
Instruct parents and child on 1. refraining from scratching 2. frequent handwashing 3. use of separate washcloth and towel 4. laundering linen in hot water 5. inspecting all family members for infection	These preventive techniques reduce the spread of organisms.
Instruct parents on administration of oral antibiotics.	Antibiotics may be needed to treat minor infection not responding to topicals and major infections. Penicillin VK, erythromycin, or dicloxacillin may be ordered for a 10-day course. Exudate is contagious for first 48 hr of treatment.
Provide suggestions for age appropriate diversional activities.	

▼

DISCHARGE PLANNING/CONTINUITY OF CARE

- Instruct parents to return in 3 days if significant improvement is not seen.
- Child may return to school after 48 hr of antibiotic therapy or, if not taking antibiotics, after vesicles are healed.
- Refer to dermatologist, immunologist, or nephrologist if needed.

LEAD POISONING

Michele Knoll Puzas, RNC, MHPE

Lead poisoning in children most often occurs as a result of long-term ingestion of substance containing lead salts. Lead salts bind with erythrocytes and interfere with heme production. Tissue damage and anemia occur when the rate of ingestion exceeds the rate of excretion by the kidneys, alimentary tract, and sweat glands.

ETIOLOGIES

- Pica behaviors in young children
- Improper food preparation
- Addictive behaviors

CLINICAL MANIFESTATIONS

- Pallor
- Headache
- Vomiting
- Irritability
- Drowsiness
- Seizures
- Peripheral nerve palsy
- Coma

CLINICAL/DIAGNOSTIC FINDINGS

- Anemia
- Lead level > 15 μg/dL
- Increased reticulocytes
- Proteinuria

▼

NURSING DIAGNOSIS: ALTERED TISSUE PERFUSION

Related To
- Decreased hemoglobin
- Decreased hematocrit
- Increased lead level

Defining Characteristics
Pallor
Cyanosis
Tachycardia
Fatigue
Irritability
Sleepiness
Weakness

Patient Outcome
Child's serum lead level will be < 15 μg/dL.

Nursing Interventions	Rationales
Assess for lead poisoning if child presents with symptoms (pallor, cyanosis, behavioral changes, fatigue, etc.) unexplained by organic or other etiology.	Lead poisoning has devastating/ lasting consequences if undiagnosed or untreated.
Determine access to lead-containing materials: 1. paint, old paint chips 2. batteries 3. color print newspapers 4. pet food 5. foods prepared or served in improperly glazed pottery 6. acidic foods/liquids served from lead crystal	
Assess child's developmental level.	Infants and toddlers are more likely to ingest foreign objects. School-age and adolescent children are more likely involved in glue/paint/gasoline sniffing. Some glues/gasolines still contain lead.

Nursing Interventions	Rationales
Determine food preparation/serving practices. Explain to parents that cracked or unglazed pottery, lead crystal baby bottles, pewter, and other similar items should not be used in cooking or food service.	
Obtain blood for lead level.	Lead level is a determining factor in selection of treatment regimen.
Explain treatment plan to parents:	
1. Children with significant symptomatology and high lead levels (> 45 µg/dL) will require hospitalization for chelation therapy.	Significant anemia and lead poisoning result in potentially life-threatening events: hypoxia, increased intracranial pressure, seizures, and coma.
2. Children with minor symptoms and moderate lead levels (15–45 µg/dL), but whose home environment is questionable, may require hospitalization.	Hospitalization is necessary to prevent further ingestion and ensure adequate treatment until home environment can be evaluated.
3. Children with minor symptoms and low lead level may be considered for outpatient chelation therapy.	
4. Local board of health or department of family services will be notified of lead poisoning.	Child's environment will be evaluated for lead-bearing materials so that removal can occur.

▼

NURSING DIAGNOSIS: KNOWLEDGE DEFICIT

Related To
- Unfamiliarity with poison prevention, effects of lead poisoning, chelation therapy
- No previous experience

Defining Characteristics
Stated lack of knowledge
Questions
Behavior inappropriate for situation

Patient Outcomes

- Parent will follow through with child's therapy and follow-up.
- Child's environment will be lead free.
- Child will not ingest/inhale lead salts.

Nursing Interventions	Rationales
Assess parent's understanding of diagnosis and its cause. Assess child/adolescent's understanding of relationship of behaviors to diagnosis and consequences.	
Explain lead poisoning and potential consequences.	Chronic ingestion can lead to mental retardation as well as other pathologies.
Explain the importance of controlling lead in the child's environment.	Poisoning will recur.
Explain chelation therapy: 1. Calcium disodium edetate (EDTA), given intramuscularly (IM), increases urinary excretion of free lead. 2. Dimercaprol (BAL, British Anti-Lewisite), effective in removing lead from nervous system, also is given IM.	
3. A combination therapy of EDTA and BAL may be prescribed.	This is for improved chelation of lead and decreased side effects resulting from chelators (nephrotoxicity, hypocalcemia).
4. Succimer (Chemet) is an *oral* chelating agent that may be prescribed. The entire 19-day course must be consumed.	This is used to lessen lead level effectively and prevent rebound rise in serum lead level.
Explain need for hospitalization, if necessary.	
Discuss importance of follow-up appointments and lead screening.	

▼

DISCHARGE PLANNING/CONTINUITY OF CARE

- Notify local agencies involved in child care: Board of Health, Family and Children's Services.
- Refer to social worker and arrange visiting nurse if needed.
- Follow up every 1–2 weeks to evaluate serum lead level, urinary function, and neurological status until stable.
- Notify school/teacher of any lasting neurological damage. Arrange for testing and alternative schooling if needed.

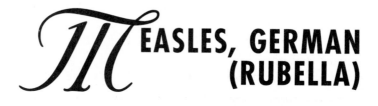

MEASLES, GERMAN (RUBELLA)

Ellen Polite, RN

German measles is a contagious viral disease, typically regarded as a childhood illness, that can be contracted by anyone not adequately immunized. If contracted during the first trimester of pregnancy, it can cause serious congenital injuries, including growth and mental retardation, deafness, and eye and heart defects. Infants born with rubella can be contagious for months.

ETIOLOGY

Infection with rubivirus

CLINICAL MANIFESTATIONS

Prodromal stage (may not be evident in children)
- Headache
- Anorexia, malaise
- Lymphadenopathy
- Low-grade fever
- Coryza, cough, sore throat
- Mild conjunctivitis

Rash
- Pinkish red maculopapular rash begins on face, spreads downward; usually gone in 3 days.

CLINICAL/DIAGNOSTIC FINDINGS

None

▼

NURSING DIAGNOSIS: INFECTION
Related To rubella virus

Defining Characteristics
See Clinical Manifestations

Patient Outcome
Child will be isolated during period of communicability.

Nursing Interventions	Rationales
Assess for signs of infection.	
Determine when rash first appeared.	Infection is communicable for at least 5 days after appearance of rash.
Explain that disease poses little risk to the child but can be extremely dangerous to a fetus during the first trimester.	
Isolate child from pregnant women and all unimmunized or immunosuppressed persons.	
Encourage immunization of all children and women of childbearing age.	Damage done in utero is devastating and lifelong. This possibility can be eradicated only with immunization.
Instruct parents to administer ibuprofen or acetaminophen to alleviate child's fever and discomfort.	

▼

DISCHARGE PLANNING/CONTINUITY OF CARE

- Follow-up is necessary only if complications are suspected (uncontrolled fever, arthritis, encephalitis, purpura).
- Refer to local Board of Health for help with immunizations if needed.

MEASLES (RUBEOLA)

Michele Knoll Puzas, RNC, MHPE

Measles is a viral disease, spread by contact with respiratory secretions, blood, or urine of infected persons, that produces more severe symptomatology than rubella but is less dangerous. It does not have a teratogenic effect on the fetus. It is contagious for approximately 5 days after rash appears.

ETIOLOGY

Infection with paramyxovirus

CLINICAL MANIFESTATIONS

Prodromal stage
- Anorexia
- Lymphadenopathy
- Fever
- Malaise

Followed by
- Coryza
- Conjunctivitis with photophobia
- Cough
- Koplik spots

Followed by
- Erythematous maculopapular rash on face

Rash
- Spreads downward
- Gradually becomes brownish, then disappears
- Fine desquamation can occur where rash is extensive

CLINICAL/DIAGNOSTIC FINDINGS

None required

▼

NURSING DIAGNOSIS: PAIN

Related To infectious process

Defining Characteristics
Verbalized discomfort
Irritability
Photophobia

Patient Outcomes
Child will verbalize or demonstrate increased comfort as evidenced by
- less rubbing of eyes.
- less irritability.

Nursing Interventions	Rationales
Assess for pain.	
Assess for coryza, conjunctivitis, photophobia, Koplik spots, and rash.	Severity of symptoms affects amount of pain.
Assess cornea for ulceration.	Corneal ulceration resulting from infection and/or rubbing may need more aggressive treatment or referral.
Explain comfort measures parents can provide at home:	
1. Use cool mist vaporizer.	Keeps skin and mucous membranes moist, decreases irritation.
2. Protect skin around nares with Vaseline or similar product.	
3. Dim lights.	
4. Clean eyes with warm saline solution to remove crusts and secretions.	
5. Provide tepid baths.	
6. Administer analgesic.	

▼

NURSING DIAGNOSIS: HYPERTHERMIA

Related To infectious process

Defining Characteristics
Body temperature > 38°C (100.4°F)
Diaphoresis
Hot, flushed skin
Decreased urine output
Seizure

Patient Outcomes
The child's temperature will
• not spike > 40°C (104°F).
• be ≤ 38°C (100.4°F).

Nursing Interventions	Rationales
Assess temperature.	
Inform parents that temperature spikes may occur around the 4th or 5th day of illness.	
Instruct parent to 1. administer ibuprofen or acetaminophen.	
2. provide tepid baths, but avoid chilling.	Chilling and shivering cause increased heat production.
3. measure temperature every 8 hr or more frequently if fever is suspected. 4. call health care provider or return to office if temperature cannot be controlled.	
5. observe for seizure activity, especially when spiking or if child has experienced seizures in the past.	Some infants are prone to febrile seizures.

▼

DISCHARGE PLANNING/CONTINUITY OF CARE

- Encourage routine immunization of others in household.
- Refer to local Board of Health.
- Discuss signs and symptoms of otitis media, pneumonia, and encephalitis requiring immediate follow-up.
- Follow up in 1–2 weeks or sooner if complications are suspected.

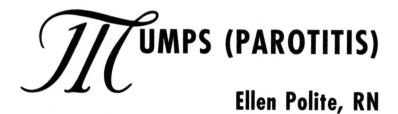UMPS (PAROTITIS)

Ellen Polite, RN

Mumps is an acute viral disease that usually affects unimmunized children between 5 and 15 years of age, but may occur at any age. Usually occurring in late winter and early spring, this highly communicable disease is spread through droplets or direct contact with saliva of infected person.

ETIOLOGY

Infection with paramyxovirus

CLINICAL MANIFESTATIONS

Prodromal stage
- Headache
- Fever
- Malaise
- Anorexia
- Earache

Followed by
- Parotitis
- Pain
- Tenderness

CLINICAL/DIAGNOSTIC FINDINGS

None required

▼

NURSING DIAGNOSIS: PAIN

Related To infectious process

Defining Characteristics
Verbal statement of pain
Guarding behavior on exam
Crying
Restlessness
Seeking out caregiver/parent (clinging)

Patient Outcome
Child will verbalize or demonstrate increased comfort as evidenced by ability to eat, drink, and sleep without difficulty.

Nursing Interventions	Rationales
Assess parotid glands.	Swelling, pain, tenderness may be bilateral or unilateral.
Assess submaxillary and sublingual glands, as well as testicles in the male, for signs of swelling or infection.	Other sites of pain/swelling may occur.
Assess neurological status, especially for increasing headache, irritability, and vomiting.	These symptoms may indicate meningoencephalitis.
Explain disease process to parents/child.	
Instruct parents to 1. limit child's activities and encourage rest. 2. administer acetaminophen or ibuprofen for pain, fever, and irritability.	
3. provide soft foods and plenty of liquids.	Chewing exacerbates ear pain.
4. apply warm or cool compresses around neck.	

▼

NURSING DIAGNOSIS: INFECTION
Related To viral disease

Defining Characteristics
Parotitis
Orchitis
Pain
Fever

Patient Outcome

Child will be isolated during period of communicability.

Nursing Interventions	Rationales
Determine onset of symptoms.	Virus may be communicable from 1 week prior to 1½ weeks after parotid swelling.
Explain necessity for isolation from susceptible individuals.	Disease can cause serious and permanent complications: 1. deafness 2. encephalitis 3. arthritis 4. myocarditis 5. hepatitis 6. sterility in adult males

▼

DISCHARGE PLANNING/CONTINUITY OF CARE

- Follow up in 1–2 weeks or sooner if signs of complication develop.
- Encourage immunization of others at risk.
- Refer to local Board of Health for help with immunizations if needed.

*O*TITIS MEDIA

Michele Knoll Puzas, RNC, MHPE

Otitis media (middle ear infection) is a fairly common disorder in young children as a result of the horizontal position of the eustachian tube, the frequency of tube blockage, and the inappropriate opening of the tube to the pharynx.

ETIOLOGIES

- Upper respiratory infections
- Cleft palate
- Adenoiditis or respiratory allergy

CLINICAL MANIFESTATIONS

- Pain
- Irritability
- Fever
- Ear drainage
- Ear pulling/rubbing
- Mild hearing loss
- Fluid behind tympanic membrane
- Red, bulging membrane
- Decreased membrane movement

CLINICAL/DIAGNOSTIC FINDINGS

None required

▼

NURSING DIAGNOSIS: INFECTION

Related To
- *Haemophilus influenzae*
- Beta-hemolytic streptococci
- *Branhamella catarrhalis*

Defining Characteristics

Pain in ear
Ear pulling/rubbing
Fever
Irritability
Diarrhea
Vomiting
Discharge from ear
Outer ear red, warm, tender

Patient Outcome

The child will be afebrile and pain free.

Nursing Interventions	Rationales
Assess for history of upper respiratory infections, ear infections, allergies, and cleft palate.	
Assess for fever and rhinorrhea. Assess tympanic membrane for 1. discharge, perforation 2. fullness 3. redness 4. decreased mobility	Symptomatology provides a clinical picture on which treatment will be based.
Instruct parents in the administration of antipyretic and antibiotics. Antibiotics of choice include: amoxicillin, Augmentin, Bactrim, erythromycin, and Ceclor.	Understanding of treatment regimen improves compliance.
Instruct parents to continue full 10-day course of antibiotics even if the child is significantly improved (usually within 24 hr).	Completing the course of antibiotics is necessary to control infection and prevent recurrence.

Nursing Interventions	Rationales
Explain the causes of otitis media and preventive measures that may be helpful. 1. Do not feed child in supine position. 2. Do not give child a bottle to fall asleep with while lying in crib. 3. Do not prop bottles.	Swallowing in the supine position increases the chance of fluids from the pharynx being drawn into the eustachian tube.
Encourage parents to provide fluids that the child prefers.	Oral fluids will help control fever.

▼

NURSING DIAGNOSIS: PAIN

Related To erythema and swelling of the middle ear with blockage of the eustachian tube

Defining Characteristics
Crying, irritability
Ear pulling/rubbing
Difficulty feeding
Verbalized pain

Patient Outcomes
• The child will verbalize adequate pain control.
• The infant will be calm and will feed easily.

Nursing Interventions	Rationales
Assess level of pain.	Each person demonstrates a unique response to pain.
Identify previously used pain control measures and effectivness.	
Instruct parents on pain control: 1. oral analgesia (acetaminophen) 2. ear drops (Auralgan) 3. warm packs to ears	A variety of interventions may be required to relieve discomfort optimally.
Instruct parents on administration of antihistamine/decongestant.	This may be prescribed to decrease blockage in eustachian tubes.

▼

DISCHARGE PLANNING/CONTINUITY OF CARE

- Instruct parents to return if
  - no improvement is seen 24 hr after beginning antibiotics.
  - there is a reaction to medications.
- Return visit should occur in 10–14 days.
- Refer to otolaryngologist for repeated infections or persistent hearing loss.
- Prophylactic antibiotic maintenance may be necessary to control chronic, frequent infection.

$\mathscr{P}$EDICULOSIS CAPITIS (HEAD LICE)

Michele Knoll Puzas, RNC, MHPE

Pediculus humanis capitis is an ectoparasite that infests the scalp. Eggs (nits) are attached to hair shafts, hatch in 10 days, and mature in 2 weeks. The insects bite, inject digestive juices, and feed on blood. Bites and excrement cause severe itching.

ETIOLOGY

Infestation resulting from use of contaminated objects (brushes, combs, hats, pillows) or direct contact.

CLINICAL MANIFESTATIONS

Itching/scratching

CLINICAL/DIAGNOSTIC FINDINGS

- Visible lice on scalp/behind ears
- Visible nits on hair

▼

NURSING DIAGNOSIS: HIGH RISK FOR IMPAIRED SKIN INTEGRITY

Risk Factors
- Insect infestation/bites
- Pruritus/scratching

Patient Outcomes
- Child's scalp/hair will be free from lice and nits.

- Sources of infestation will be treated.
- Secondary scalp infections will not occur.

Nursing Interventions	Rationales
Inspect scalp and hair shafts for evidence of lice and nits (or nit cases).	
Assess for skin damage and pyoderma.	Damaged skin increases the risk of infection.
Show the parent what lice and nits look like.	Parents will need to inspect child and other family members periodically.
Instruct parent to	
1. Obtain pediculicidal shampoo or creme rinse. • Apply shampoo to child's scalp and hair, closely following product directions. • Keep out of child's eyes.	Kwell (lindane) can cause toxic reactions if used improperly (contact dermatitis or central nervous system toxicity). Kwell should not be used by pregnant women.
• Use fine-tooth comb (sometimes provided with product) to remove lice/nits. Long hair can be brushed out first, then combed in sections.	Nits and nit cases adhere to hair shafts. A brush or wide toothed comb will not slide closely enough to hair shaft to remove adherent nits.
2. Clean all contaminated brushes, combs, barrettes, and the like with pediculicide. Hair equipment also can be boiled for at least 10 min to kill insects and eggs.	
3. Wash all clothing, hats, and linens that the child has used in hot water. Unwashable items can be tightly bagged for about 4 days.	Lice die in 3 days without nourishment.
4. Consider new pillows, if not washable.	
5. Vacuum mattress, carpeting, and other furniture. Discard vacuum bag.	Ova may be dormant for 4–5 weeks. Hatched nymphs must feed in 24 hr; lice can crawl.

Nursing Interventions	Rationales
6. Inspect other family members for lice and treat accordingly.	
7. Inform school/day care provider.	School epidemics have occurred; authorities should be informed so any classroom measures can be implemented.
8. Reapply pediculicidal (Kwell) agent/shampoo as directed. Creme rinse (Nix) may not need reapplication.	Missed nits will hatch within two weeks. Nix creme rinse's ovicidal effect is active for 14 days.
9. Apply Vaseline to eyelashes/eyebrows with adherent nits.	After 24 hr the nit will wipe away more easily.

▼

NURSING DIAGNOSIS: HIGH RISK FOR SITUATIONAL LOW SELF-ESTEEM

Risk Factors
- Diagnosis of pediculosis
- Verbalized shame or guilt
- Knowledge deficit

Patient Outcomes
Child and parent will deal with situation and maintain self-esteem as evidenced by
- verbal understanding of cause.
- follow-through with treatment plan.
- verbal statement of positive self-esteem.

Nursing Interventions	Rationales
Explain that lice are spread easily and rapidly, and infestation is unrelated to cleanliness or economics.	
Encourage parent to remain calm and treat the situation in a "matter-of-fact" manner.	The child will be better able to handle the situation if the parent does not overreact.

Nursing Interventions	Rationales
Discourage radical haircuts and head shaving.	Radical changes in how the child looks affects his/her vision of self and his/her relationship with peers. With medicinal control such as Kwell, Rid, or R & C shampoo, severe haircuts are no longer necessary.

▼

DISCHARGE PLANNING/CONTINUITY OF CARE

- Encourage all family members to be examined for pediculosis.
- Each person with infestation must be treated or reinfestation of others will occur.
- Follow up in 1 month or sooner if needed.
- Refer to dermatologist for additional scalp infections.
- Refer to social service if reinfestations occur repeatedly.

PERTUSSIS (WHOOPING COUGH)

Barb Hartz, RN, MS, CNP

Pertussis is an acute upper respiratory infection seen in unimmunized infants and children. This infection, usually seen in the spring and summer, can cause severe complications, including pneumonia, atelectasis, emphysema, otitis, cerebral edema, intracranial hemorrhage, and seizures.

ETIOLOGY

Infection with *Bordetella pertussis* bacillus contained in respiratory secretions.

CLINICAL MANIFESTATIONS

Catarrhal stage
- Upper respiratory infection symptoms for 1–2 weeks
- Low-grade fever
- Worsening nighttime cough

Paroxysmal stage
- Dry hacking cough, increasing in severity
- High-pitched whooping sound on inspiration
- Expulsion of thick mucus

Convalescent stage
- Lasts 4–6 weeks
- Residual cough

CLINICAL/DIAGNOSTIC FINDINGS

- Leukocytosis
- Positive sputum culture

▼

NURSING DIAGNOSIS: INEFFECTIVE AIRWAY CLEARANCE

Related To
- Thick mucus in airway
- Infectious process

Defining Characteristics
Dry, repetitive cough
Inspirational whoop
Facial flushing or cyanosis
Expulsion of mucus plug
Vomiting mucus
Cyanosis
Increased respiratory rate

Patient Outcomes
The child will have
- less frequent paroxysmal coughing.
- less severe episodes of coughing.

Nursing Interventions	Rationales
Assess for airway obstruction.	Increasing obstruction is life threatening.
Assess severity of paroxysmal coughing.	Prolonged or frequent paroxysmal episodes may require hospitalization to prevent/treat anoxia and its complications. Children < 1 year old are at greatest risk.
Explain disease process to parents.	
Assure parents and child that, although the coughing episodes are frightening, they usually are not dangerous. Discuss home care, including	
1. providing calm physical and emotional support during coughing episodes.	Obvious anxiety in the caregiver can heighten the child's fear and anxiety.
2. controlling external stimuli such as dust and smoke.	Dust, smoke, noise, physical exertion, and temperature changes can stimulate coughing.

Nursing Interventions	Rationales
3. preventing spread of infection.	
4. administering antibiotics and antipyretics.	Antibiotics may be ordered to reduce risk of contagion, as well as risk of secondary bacterial infection.
5. maintaining bed rest or quiet play.	
6. humidifying room air.	

▼

NURSING DIAGNOSIS: FLUID VOLUME DEFICIT

Related To
- Vomiting
- Poor appetite/exhaustion
- Insensible water loss

Defining Characteristics
Weight loss
Decreased urine output
Dry mucous membranes
Increased temperature
Sunken eyes, fontanel
Weakness/sleepiness

Patient Outcomes
The child will be able to drink and retain fluids.

Nursing Interventions	Rationales
Assess hydration.	Infants and children with significant dehydration may need immediate referral, hospitalization, and intravenous fluids.
Assess history of vomiting and ability to take food and fluids.	
Recommend small, frequent meals, with fluids available at all times.	

Nursing Interventions	Rationales
Offer food and fluids after paroxysmal spells.	After expelling mucus from airway and stomach, the child may be able to retain nutritional offerings.

▼

DISCHARGE PLANNING/CONTINUITY OF CARE

- Teach parents how to aspirate mucus from upper airway.
- Explain symptoms requiring immediate return visit: convulsions, uncontrolled vomiting, decreased urination, unresolved cyanosis. Child may appear cyanotic during paroxysm but color should return to normal when coughing is over.
- Follow up in 1–2 weeks, depending on age and severity of symptoms. Examine for hernia and rectal prolapse on return visits.
- Isolate infected child from other young children.
- Recommend immunization of other infants, children in household.
- Refer to Visiting Nurse Association if needed.

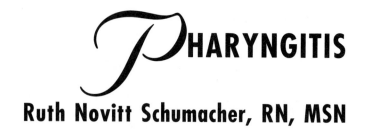

PHARYNGITIS

Ruth Novitt Schumacher, RN, MSN

Pharyngitis is an inflammation of the pharynx with pain in the throat. Its onset may be gradual, over a day or two, or abrupt.

ETIOLOGY

May be viral or bacterial

CLINICAL MANIFESTATIONS

- Fever
- Headache
- Malaise
- Dysphagia
- Throat pain
- Postnasal secretions
- Anterior cervical lymphadenopathy
- Enlarged tonsils

CLINICAL/DIAGNOSTIC FINDINGS

- Normal or slightly elevated white blood cell count
- Positive throat culture if bacterial (streptococcus)

▼

NURSING DIAGNOSIS: HYPERTHERMIA

Related To body's response to invasion of viral or bacterial antigens.

Defining Characteristics
Temperature > 38.4°C (101°F)
Chills
Diaphoresis
Dehydration
Increased heart rate
Increased respiratory rate
Irritability

Patient Outcome
Child's temperature will return to normal within 24 hr.

Nursing Interventions	Rationales
Assess temperature and history of onset.	
Assess for chills, shaking, and diaphoresis.	
Assess for signs of dehydration: 1. dry mucous membranes 2. presence/absence of tears 3. decreased and/or dark urine output 4. decreased skin turgor	
Determine history of intake of foods/fluids.	
Explain necessity of and procedure for obtaining throat culture.	
Instruct parents to:	
1. Administer antipyretics as ordered. (Do not give aspirin because of its link with Reye's syndrome).	
2. Administer antibiotics.	If a bacterial infection is confirmed, untreated streptococcal infections can lead to scarlet fever and its complications.
3. Dress child lightly.	Overdressing may cause temperature to increase.

Nursing Interventions	Rationales
Refer infants with significant dehydration to emergency room or hospital.	Infant may require intravenous fluid therapy; older children usually can be rehydrated orally when fever and pain are controlled.

▼

NURSING DIAGNOSIS: HIGH RISK FOR FLUID VOLUME DEFICIT

Risk Factors
- Reduced intake/lack of interest in eating or drinking
- Pain when drinking/eating
- Fever

Patient Outcome
Child will maintain adequate hydration.

Nursing Interventions	Rationales
Assess hydration status, including 1. mucous membranes 2. presence/absences of tears 3. skin turgor 4. urine output	
Instruct parents to administer analgesics/antipyretics.	Pain resulting from inflammation of the pharynx and anterior cervical lymph nodes as well as associated fever can prevent child from drinking adequate amounts.
Offer small amounts of preferred fluids frequently.	
Involve the child in drinking. Provide age-appropriate incentives: special bottle or cup, use of a sick cup or straws while in bed. Try a variety of fruit juices.	

▼

DISCHARGE PLANNING/CONTINUITY OF CARE

- Instruct parents on the purpose, dosage, and administration of antipyretic and antibiotic therapy. Review side effects.
- Instruct parents to call and/or see physician if child shows no improvement within 48 hr, becomes suddenly worse, or develops a rash.

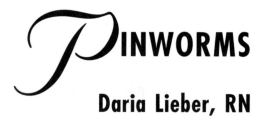

PINWORMS

Daria Lieber, RN

A parasitic infestation, pinworms (enterobiasis, oxyuriasis, scatworm) can affect any age group but place toddlers and young school-age children at highest risk because of hand-mouth activity and uncontrolled toilet habits. Pinworm is the most common parasitic disease in North America, transmitted through the fecal-oral route and inhalation of airborne eggs. Infestation occurs only in humans and cannot be contracted from pets.

ETIOLOGY

Infestation with *Enterobius vermicularis*

CLINICAL MANIFESTATIONS

- Rectal, perineal, and vaginal itching
- Excoriated skin and secondary infection resulting from scratching

CLINICAL/DIAGNOSTIC FINDINGS

Microscopic evidence of pinworms

▼

NURSING DIAGNOSIS: INFECTION

Related To presence of *Enterobius vermicularis*

Defining Characteristics
Severe perianal itching
Scratching
Excoriated skin
Crying, irritability

Patient Outcome
The child will have no evidence of eggs or pinworms on exam.

Nursing Interventions	Rationales
Examine perianal and vaginal area for evidence of scratching and secondary infection and/or pinworms.	Pinworms usually are not seen during the day; only evidence of scratching will be seen.
Recommend frequent, gentle cleansing.	This is to provide comfort and alleviate secondary infection.
Explain suspected diagnosis and specimens necessary for microscopic examination.	
Instruct parent to apply sticky side of cellulose tape to perianal folds during the night when itching occurs or in the morning on awakening.	At night, mature female pinworm migrates from the intestine to deposit eggs on the perianal area and perineum. Migration into the vagina also occurs. Ova and parasites will stick to the tape.
Instruct to collect pinworm specimen using a commercially made collection device or a loop of home cellulose tape and to enclose in a plastic ziplock bag or jar.	
Instruct parent to bring specimen to lab or doctor's office. A stool specimen also may be requested for this purpose.	Specimen is needed for microscopic examination.
Explain medication prescribed to destroy parasite: • Vermox (mebendazole), 1 tablet given twice daily for 3 days, or • Antiminth (pyrantel pamoate), given 10 mg/kg, not to exceed 1 g. Dosage may be repeated in 2 weeks.	Consistent blood levels are needed to prevent reinfection.

▼

NURSING DIAGNOSIS: KNOWLEDGE DEFICIT

Related To
• New diagnosis
• Unfamiliarity with treatment plan and procedures to prevent infestation

Defining Characteristics
Verbalized lack of understanding
Questions

Patient Outcome
Child will be adequately treated and reinfestation will not occur.

Nursing Interventions	Rationales
Assess parents' understanding of parasitic infection and its transmission and eradication.	Parent must follow through with eradication in the home, or reinfestation will occur.
Explain 1. Medication and dosage.	
2. Rationale for treating other family members, if this is prescribed.	Family treatment may be prescribed if reinfestation has occurred. Medication is not recommended for children under two years or pregnant women.
3. Necessity for scrupulous hand washing, especially after toileting and before meals or food preparation.	
4. Need for teaching good hygiene practices to children.	
5. Importance of cleaning technique for child's bedding, floor, furniture, and clothing: • Floor and furniture should be vacuumed or washed. • Mattress should be vacuumed. • Child's linen, blankets, and clothing (esp. pajamas and underwear) should be machine washed in hot water.	Measures are required to kill all existing ova before hatching.
Discuss caring for the infected child: 1. Scrub child's hands and fingernails; cut fingernails short.	Ova adhere under fingernails.
2. Discourage thumbsucking and nail biting. Give child alternative (pacifier, pretzel, cracker, etc.).	

Nursing Interventions	**Rationales**
3. Dress child with underwear and pajamas at night.	This is to contain migration and spread of ova and parasites.
4. Remove underwear/pajamas in the bathtub and shower child every morning with careful rinsing of the perineum/perianal areas.	
5. Launder underwear, pajamas, and linen daily. Do not shake out.	Shaking will cause ova to become airborne. Ova can remain viable without human host for days.
6. Dress child in clean underwear and clothing.	
Reassure parents that pinworms can be controlled and there are no significant systemic complications.	Rarely, symptoms of appendicitis occur.

▼

DISCHARGE PLANNING/CONTINUITY OF CARE

- Follow up in 3 weeks if symptoms return. Treatment may need to be repeated.
- Refer
  - children under 2 years to pediatrician/infectious disease specialist.
  - any pregnant family members to gynecologist.

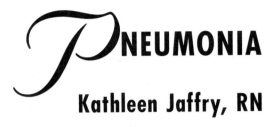

PNEUMONIA

Kathleen Jaffry, RN

Pneumonia is an acute inflammation of the lungs. Lobar pneumonia involves entire lobe or lobes of one or both lungs. Bronchopneumonia involves terminal bronchioles and lobules. Interstitial pneumonia involves interstitium of alveolar walls and peribronchial and interlobular tissues.

ETIOLOGIES

- Bacterial—streptococcus, staphylococcus, *Haemophilus influenzae*, and *Diplococcus pneumoniae*
- Viral—respiratory syncytial virus, flu, rhinovirus, and adenovirus.
- Mycoplasmas—*mycoplasma pneumoniae*
- Foreign body—aspiration
- Fungal (rarely)—histomycosis or other fungi, usually secondary to other illness

CLINICAL MANIFESTATIONS

- Severe chills
- Fever
- Headache
- Cough
- Chest pain
- Abnormal chest sounds
  - viral: few rhonchi, fine rales
  - mycoplasma: fine crepitant rales, possible consolidation
  - bacterial: shallow respirations, pleural effusion, rapid consolidation

CLINICAL/DIAGNOSTIC FINDINGS

- Positive chest films
- Positive sputum culture

▼

NURSING DIAGNOSIS: INEFFECTIVE AIRWAY CLEARANCE

Related To congestion of lobes and decreased lung expansion

Defining Characteristics

Abnormal breath sounds
Cough (effective or ineffective)
Dyspnea
Fatigue
Cyanosis
Change in respiratory status
Infiltrate on chest x-ray

Patient Outcomes

- Child's airway will be freed of secretions.
- Child's lung sounds will be normal.

Nursing Interventions	Rationales
Assess breath sounds.	Rales and bronchial breath sounds may be heard over affected areas.
Assess respiratory rate, depth, and character.	Shallow, splinted respirations are common.
Assess use of accessory muscles.	This may indicate severe hypoxemia.
Assess sputum: amount and color.	If child is unable to produce sputum, transtracheal aspiration may be required.
Assess for change in orientation, cyanosis.	Indicates severe hypoxia requiring immediate treatment.
Explain all diagnostic tests:	
1. chest x-ray	This provides information on the site of involvement
2. pulse oximetry	Excellent, noninvasive test of oxygenation.
3. sputum for culture/Gram's stain	This provides diagnostic information on type of organism present, which is needed to guide therapy.

Nursing Interventions	Rationales
4. complete blood count	Leukocytosis usually is evident in pneumonia.
5. blood culture	This should be done if bacterial infection is suspected.
Explain need to drink plenty of fluids, at least 6–8 glasses daily.	Improved, adequate hydration helps to liquify secretions and ease breathing.
Encourage patient to deep breathe. Explain breathing games that can be used with the young child: blowing bubbles, balloons, Three Little Pigs.	This is to maintain full lung expansion and adequate ventilation.
Encourage child to cough.	This prevents retained secretions, which compromise gas exchange.
Control cough if it is not productive.	This can cause both hypoxemia and added fatigue.
Explain need to reduce activity, especially during febrile period.	Adequate rest is needed for recovery and to prevent relapse.
Explain that fatigue and weakness may persist after recovery, and therefore child should return slowly to normal activity level.	
Explain importance of taking the full course of antibiotics as prescribed.	Antibiotics may be prescribed for child with viral illness to prevent secondary bacterial infection.

▼

NURSING DIAGNOSIS: INFECTION

Related To invading bacteria, virus, fungus

Defining Characteristics
Fever
Chills
Dyspnea
Chest pain

Patient Outcomes
- The child will be able to breathe without dyspnea and pain.
- Child/parents will verbalize understanding of treatment plan.

Nursing Interventions	Rationales
Assess respiratory status.	Most pneumonias can be treated on an outpatient basis. However, severe dyspnea may warrant hospitalization.
Determine temperature and onset of chills and fever.	
Assess for pain on respiration/ coughing.	Pleuritic chest pain may impair adequate ventilation; appropriate therapy is indicated.
Explain type of pneumonia child has and specific treatment.	
Instruct family in home care measures:	
1. acetaminophen	Needed to control both fever and pain.
2. antibiotics	To control infection and prevent relapse.
3. cough suppressant if indicated	Unproductive coughing may increase pain and hypoxia, and exhaust child.
4. room humidifier	To loosen secretions, ease breathing, and maintain hydration.
5. plenty of oral fluids	Fever and increased respiration can lead to dehydration.
Explain need for small frequent meals of desired, tolerated foods, especially those high in protein/ carbohydrates.	Child may be unable to tolerate large meals because of difficulty breathing and fatigue. Small frequent meals will maintain nutrition/caloric intake.
Encourage rest and quiet activities.	This reduces metabolic and respiratory demands. Quiet activities are less likely to cause coughing, dyspnea, and pain.

Nursing Interventions	Rationales
Explain reasons for hospitalization if indicated.	Severe illness with bacterial infection may require intravenous antibiotics and oxygen therapy. Infants with respiratory syncytial virus are at risk for respiratory failure and may require medicated inhalation therapy (Ribavirin) and intravenous hydration. Also, any child who has developed complications (empyema, pneumothorax, septicemia), who is immunosuppressed, or whose pneumonia is secondary to another condition will require close observation and aggressive treatment.

▼

DISCHARGE PLANNING/CONTINUITY OF CARE

- Follow-up is determined based on age of child and severity of illness.
- Schedule return in at least 1 week, sooner for infants or severely ill child.
- Instruct parents to call/return if no improvement or worsening of symptoms is noted.
- Repeat chest films in 2–4 weeks if breath sounds continue to be abnormal.

SCARLET FEVER

Bernadette Keller, RN, BSN

Scarlet fever is an early childhood infectious disease usually affecting 6–12-year-olds. The incubation period is 2–4 days. Complications from scarlet fever include the development of acute glomerulonephritis or acute rheumatic fever.

ETIOLOGY

Group A beta-hemolytic streptococcus infection of throat or skin

CLINICAL MANIFESTATIONS

- High fever
- Vomiting
- Headache
- Chills
- Tonsils become red and enlarged, and covered with exudate
- Strawberry tongue
- Generalized rash may appear within 12 hr
- Desquamation

CLINICAL/DIAGNOSTIC FINDINGS

- Throat culture positive for group A beta-hemolytic streptococcus
- Positive antistreptolysin-O titer
- Leukocytosis

▼

NURSING DIAGNOSIS: INFECTION

Related To presence of group A beta-hemolytic streptococci in respiratory tract

Defining Characteristics

Fever
Sore throat (red, swollen tonsils/pharynx)
Fine red rash (appears within 48 hr of fever and sore throat)
Strawberry tongue
Exudate on tonsils

Patient Outcome

The child will have decreased temperature and throat pain 48 hr after initiating antibiotics.

Nursing Interventions	Rationales
Assess for exposure to strep pharyngitis.	Strep pharyngitis is highly contagious.
Assess for defining characteristics.	
Swab throat for strep culture, perform in-office strep test if possible.	
Explain importance of antibiotic therapy: penicillin G usually is ordered; penicillin V or erythromycin also are effective.	A 10-day course of antibiotics is required to arrest infection. Infection will not be controlled, symptoms will return, and there may be an increased risk for complications of scarlet fever if antibiotics are halted earlier than prescribed. Intramuscular penicillin may be necessary if there is a problem with compliance.
Instruct parent and child on home isolation strategies: 1. no sharing of cups, utensils, food 2. use of disposable cups/plates 3. keep other children away for the first 24 hr of antibiotic therapy 4. consider changing toothbrushes	The disease is transmitted through nasopharyngeal secretions from an infected individual or their articles.

▼

NURSING DIAGNOSIS: PAIN

Related To infectious process

Defining Characteristics
Throat pain
Itching with rash
Skin tenderness with desquamation
Abdominal pain

Patient Outcomes
The child's pain will be controlled as evidenced by
• decreased complaints of pain.
• improved food/fluid intake.

Nursing Interventions	Rationales
Assess condition of pharynx and tonsils. Assess skin.	Having a baseline makes it easier to observe changes to treatment.
Assess hydration.	Dry mucous membranes increase pain.
Instruct parents to 1. provide acetaminophen to control pain (older children may use ibuprofen). 2. provide soothing foods/fluids that are easy to swallow (popsicles, nonacidic juices, gelatins, ices, sherbets). 3. provide throat lozenges for the older child (risk of airway obstruction in young child). 4. maintain antibiotic therapy for full course even if child feels better in a few days.	

▼

DISCHARGE PLANNING/CONTINUITY OF CARE

• Instruct parents to return or call if
  – fever and pain persist past 48 hr of antibiotic therapy

    – child is unable to take antibiotic or adverse reaction occurs
- Follow-up should be scheduled after completion of antibiotic therapy.
- Immediate medical attention should be sought if symptoms of complications occur (usually 7–14 days after initial treatment), including
  - decreased urinary output
  - dark urine
  - anorexia
  - abdominal pain
  - fever
  - headache
  - joint pains
- Refer for cardiac, infectious disease, or renal consult.

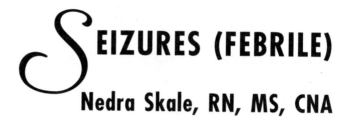

SEIZURES (FEBRILE)
Nedra Skale, RN, MS, CNA

Febrile seizures are classified as simple or complex. Simple seizures are short in duration without post-ictal neurological changes. Complex seizures usually have focal findings that last longer than 15 min, and there are transient neurological findings after the seizure. These seizures also may recur with the same illness. The risk of epilepsy is higher in children who have features of complex febrile seizures. An abnormal developmental or neurological state also causes predisposition to epilepsy. In normal children febrile seizures have no adverse impact on developmental and intellectual functioning. One third of children who have a febrile seizure will have recurrences, but recurrence does not increase the risk of epilepsy.

ETIOLOGIES

- Rapid rise in temperature secondary to infection, dehydration, or other cause
- Idiopathic (4%)

CLINICAL MANIFESTATIONS

- Mild illness: a simple seizure without any postseizure alteration in mental status
- Moderate illness: complex seizure without any postseizure alteration in mental status
- Severe illness: complex seizure with alteration of baseline mental status

CLINICAL/DIAGNOSTIC FINDINGS

Not required for diagnosis

▼

NURSING DIAGNOSIS: HIGH RISK FOR INJURY

Risk Factors
- Involuntary, random movements
- Postictal state
- Lack of control, self-protective behaviors/reflexes

Patient Outcomes
The child will
- have his/her airway protected to prevent atelectasis, infection, and stasis of air and secretions in the lungs.
- be prevented from injuring himself/herself.

Nursing Interventions	Rationales
Obtain an accurate history of the seizure activity.	
Measure and record baseline vital signs (temperature, pulse, respiratory rate, blood pressure).	
Note focal neurological deficits and signs of meningeal irritation (bulging fontanel, lethargy, nuchal rigidity, positive Kernig's sign or Brudzinski's sign).	Children with initial complex febrile seizures require a workup to identify a bacterial meningitis (3%), a viral meningitis/encephalitis (9%), or a metabolic disorder (5%). Workup for simple seizures is not necessary because of the low incidence of meningitis (0.6%) and metabolic disorders (0.9%).
Determine predisposing illness, infection (meningitis, otitis, shigella, and roseola are common). Assess the child's degree of illness. Assess hydrational state and hemodynamic state.	More assertive medical interventions may be necessary to control illness and seizures.
Assess the child's potential for injury.	

Nursing Interventions	Rationales
Provide instructions on safety precautions:	
1. If the child is standing, ease the child to the floor. Support the child's head and gently restrain his/her hands to prevent injury from violent movements against the floor.	
2. Move away from the child any objects that he/she may strike during the seizure (furniture).	
3. Assess the child for respiratory distress during and after the seizure.	
4. Turn the child to his/her side, clear mouth of secretions.	This is to establish and maintain an adequate airway.
5. Restrict child's activities as needed.	Child may be more accepting if approached in a positive way, in terms of what *can* be done rather than what *cannot* be done.
6. Instruct the family that reduction of the body temperature by the use of conductive or evaporative cooling and the use of an antipyrexic is an early preventive measure in the event of a fever caused by infection.	Febrile seizures usually accompany upper respiratory or gastrointestinal infections. The fever usually exceeds 38°C (101.8°F) and the seizure usually occurs during the temperature rise rather than after a prolonged elevation.

NURSING DIAGNOSIS: ANXIETY/FEAR

Related To
- Unpredictability of seizures
- Seizures
- Postictal state
- Unknown complications
- Lack of knowledge

Defining Characteristics
Feelings of loss of control
Increased questioning and verbalization
Inability to comfort, irritability

Patient Outcomes

- The child and/or family will
  - use effective coping mechanisms to manage their anxiety.
  - verbalize and participate in the care needed and experience less anxiety related to fear of the unknown.
- The child will discuss his/her fears.

Nursing Interventions	Rationales
Assess the educational needs of the child and family as they relate to febrile seizures and the treatment prescribed.	
Inform the family of what a seizure is and what causes seizures: 1. Reassure them that seizures will not affect mental capacities and that the child can still attend school. 2. Reassure them that seizures will not shorten the life of the child.	
Inform the family that the child should be reared as any other normal child and not overprotected.	Behavior problems often become a more serious problem than the seizures. Delinquent behavior has been attributed to the child's reaction to parental rejection. Guilt, depression, and frustration can contribute to antisocial behavior.
Instruct the child and family on the correct administration of the treatment prescribed (phenobarbital or Depakene sometimes are prescribed).	
Instruct the child and family on the potential side effects of the drugs prescribed: 1. Phenobarbital: lethargy, unsteadiness, hyperactivity, cognitive impairment, rash. 2. Depakene: nausea, vomiting, tremor, alopecia, liver failure, pancreatitis, thrombocytopenia	

▼

DISCHARGE PLANNING/CONTINUITY OF CARE

- Encourage the family to notify the child's school of the need for medication and prompt control of fever.
- Encourage the family to obtain a Medic-Alert medallion for the child to wear.
- Refer to pediatric neurologist if needed.
- Follow-up is determined based on primary illness, fever control, and use of medications.
- Encourage family to call or return if seizures continue or worsen.

SICKLE CELL ANEMIA

JoAnn Allen, RN, BSN

Sickle cell anemia is an inherited disorder in which an abnormal hemoglobin (HbS) is produced and normal hemoglobin (HbA) is deficient or absent. Infants are born with circulating fetal hemoglobin (HbF), therefore, symptoms of the disease are not evident until after 6 months of age. Children may go undiagnosed until they experience a sickle cell crisis. Crisis develops when red blood cells (RBCs) are stressed; abnormal HbS cannot withstand decreased serum oxygen tension. The abnormal HbS causes the cell to sickle in shape. Sickled cells occlude blood vessels, causing tissue infarction and pain.

ETIOLOGY

Autosomal recessive genetic disorder

CLINICAL MANIFESTATIONS

- Failure to thrive
- Delayed growth/development
- Frequent infections

CLINICAL/DIAGNOSTIC FINDINGS

- Decreased hemoglobin, hematocrit, RBCs, hyperbilirubinemia
- Positive Sickledex
- Positive hemoglobin electrophoresis

▼

NURSING DIAGNOSIS: PAIN

Related To
- Blood vessel occlusion
- Thrombosis
- Tissue infarction
- Dehydration
- Infection

Defining Characteristics
Complaint of sudden onset of pain
Severe pain in various body parts
Joint pain
Swelling of hands/feet
Irritable
Crying

Patient Outcome
The child will verbalize pain control.

Nursing Interventions	Rationales
Determine child's/parents' perception of pain. Assess for: location, onset, duration, and intensity.	This is to assist in determining primary diagnosis and potential complications. Severe crises involving the lungs, liver, kidneys, or heart may be life threatening. Bone infarcts, splenic sequestration, and priapism also will require aggressive therapy.
Determine possible precipitating factors: infection, dehydration, stress, heat/cold exposure.	Eliminating precipitating factors is the first step in controlling pain crisis.
Arrange or obtain blood for hemoglobin electrophoresis or Sickledex.	This is necessary for definitive diagnosis, if not already known.
Determine what pain control measures have been attempted and if anything helps to alleviate the pain.	
Provide analgesic and instruction on medication administration: 1. minimal pain: plain acetaminophen	

Nursing Interventions	Rationales
2. mild to moderate pain: acetaminophen with codeine	
3. severe pain: oral demerol or morphine is available, but children in severe pain may require hospitalization for intravenous hydration and pain management.	Severe pain also is indicative of life-threatening complications: pulmonary, brain infarcts.
Provide parents information about other methods of pain control:	
1. proper positioning	To decrease stress on joints.
2. warmth (heating pad/hot water bottle)	To increase vasodilation and blood flow.
3. diversions (reading, quiet games, television)	To distract child from concentrating on pain.
4. cuddling/rocking.	
6. prayer (if appropriate)	For spiritual comfort.

▼

NURSING DIAGNOSIS: KNOWLEDGE DEFICIT

Related To new diagnosis

Defining Characteristics
Asking many questions
Verbalized concerns about home management

Patient Outcomes
Patient/parents will verbalize understanding of disease, preventive measures, and crisis management.

Nursing Interventions	**Rationales**
Determine parents' and child's understanding of disease, cause, and potential complications.	
1. Arrange genetic counseling if desired. Encourage parents to discuss genetic origin of illness with child when appropriate.	Sexually active adolescents need to understand the likelihood of passing the disease on to their children.
2. Explain the pathophysiology in terms the child/parent can understand.	
3. Discuss potential complications, including effects of crisis on major organs, resultant anemia, and susceptibility to infection.	Anemia results from impaired bone marrow function; impaired splenic function increases risk of infection.
Instruct family on how to avoid possible precipitating factors:	
1. dehydration, especially during illness, or hot weather and exercise.	Dehydration increases the viscosity of the blood and stresses the oxygen-carrying capabilities of the HbS.
2. extremes of cold and heat.	Cold causes vasoconstriction, heat causes vasodilation.
3. sudden air pressure changes, high altitudes	
4. persons with communicable illness	
Provide information on health maintenance: 1. Get adequate sleep. 2. Eat a balanced diet. 3. Drink plenty of fluids. 4. Avoid alcohol, smoking, other habits. 5. Exercise regularly, but not to extreme. 6. Keep immunizations up to date. 7. Take vitamins, supplements if prescribed. 8. Take prophylactic antibiotic, if prescribed.	

Nursing Interventions	Rationales
Inform parents and child that crises will occur and management should begin at home.	This is to prevent severe pain, tissue damage, and further anemia.
1. Identify early signs of crisis, especially in infants and toddlers, such as irritability, fever.	Infants/toddlers cannot verbalize onset of area of pain.
2. Provide oral fluids.	
3. Administer medications as prescribed.	
4. Seek medical intervention if home management is not successful.	
5. Inform teachers of school-age children about illness, special needs, and emergency contacts.	

NURSING DIAGNOSIS: HIGH RISK FOR INEFFECTIVE (COMPROMISED) FAMILY COPING

Risk Factors
- Chronic illness
- Genetic disease
- Life-style changes
- Decreased life expectancy

Patient Outcomes
Parent will demonstrate adequate coping behaviors
- Communicates effectively with child.
- Provides emotional support for child.
- Provides physical support for child.

Nursing Interventions	Rationales
Determine family's response to diagnosis, cause, and treatment plans.	Guilt may be an overriding emotion that inhibits parent's coping abilities and influences parenting.
Assess availability of support systems, extended family, school, church, and peers.	
Arrange social service referral.	Social services may be able to assist with financial and emotional stressors.

Nursing Interventions	Rationales
Assist the parents in handling child's response to illness.	Child may become withdrawn, depressed, manipulative in effort to communicate feelings of anger or inferiority.
Allow parents and child to verbalize questions, fears, and frustrations, if able.	
Clarify misconceptions, suggest options when available.	Parents may fear development of drug dependency in child, or treat the child as fragile or differently from unaffected siblings. Parents should be encouraged to allow child a life as normal as possible, including schooling, discipline, and outside activities with adequate pain control.

▼

DISCHARGE PLANNING/CONTINUITY OF CARE

- Arrange consults: hematologist, social service.
- Arrange return to office for routine well child care.
- Provide emergency phone numbers for
  - primary health care provider
  - hematologist
  - hospital/emergency room
- Provide written information concerning sickle cell disease, crisis management, pain medications, and signs and symptoms of complications.
- Encourage participation in peer support groups.

SUBSTANCE ABUSE

Kathleen Scharer, RN, MS, CS, FAAN

Substance abuse is a pattern of use of some agent(s) that alters thinking, perception, mood, or state of consciousness. The use of the substance(s) is a deviation from acceptable societal, medical, or legal norms.

ETIOLOGIES

Varied, may include
- Excessive and/or compulsive use
- Powerful immediate reinforcement
- Low self-esteem
- Dysfunctional family
- Family history of abuse
- Illness related to abuse pattern
- Inadequate coping skills
- Genetic predisposition

CLINICAL MANIFESTATIONS

- Duration of the pattern is typically > 1 month.
- Associated with impaired social, occupational, or educational functioning.
- See Nursing Diagnosis: High Risk for Injury, Risk Factors

CLINICAL/DIAGNOSTIC FINDINGS

Positive urine/blood drug screen

NURSING DIAGNOSIS: ALTERED NUTRITION—LESS THAN BODY REQUIREMENTS

Related To
- Inability to ingest or digest or absorb nutrients because of biological, psychological, or economic factors.
- Uses substances instead of ingesting nourishing foods.
- Abuses substances such as laxatives that interfere with digestion or absorption.
- Eats primarily "junk foods."
- Problems with malabsorption as a result of chronic substance abuse.
- Preoccupation with obtaining desired substance results in missed meals.
- Trades school lunches for desired substances.

Defining Characteristics
Reported inadequate food intake (less than Recommended Daily Allowance)
Lack of interest in food
Reported altered taste sensation
Body weight 20% or more under ideal for age and sex
Loss of weight with adequate food intake
Poor skin turgor
Hyponatremia, hypokalemia
Edema of extremities
Electrolyte imbalance
Cheilosis (cracks in corners of mouth)
Dermatitis—scaly
Anemias

Patient Outcomes
The child will
- consume adequate nutrients to meet Recommended Daily Allowance.
- absorb sufficient nutrients to meet metabolic needs as evidenced by weight gain and improved skin turgor and electrolyte balance.

Nursing Interventions	Rationales
Assess child's nutritional status, using a history and dietary diary kept for 1 week if possible.	When abusing substances, a child may not eat correctly.
Assess child's physical status for evidence of malnutrition.	

Nursing Interventions	Rationales
Assess child's likes and dislikes.	
Assess family's patterns of eating, types of food eaten, family meals, and knowledge of nutritional needs.	Altered nutritional status may be related to family eating patterns.
Monitor changes in status, including laboratory work, for evidence of improvements.	
Determine caloric intake required to meet metabolic requirements and establish nutritional plan, consulting with dietitian as necessary.	
Teach patient and family about the importance and components of adequate nutrition. Use multiple teaching methods.	
Teach child and family about any vitamins, minerals, or nutritional supplements ordered to improve nutritional status.	Improper usage may produce additional difficulties.
Provide anticipatory instruction about what is reasonable weight gain and how to monitor growth.	Much misinformation exists about weight and normal growth.

▼

NURSING DIAGNOSIS: HIGH RISK FOR INJURY

Risk Factors
Internal
- Biochemical, regulatory functions
  - Sensory dysfunctions
  - Integrative dysfunctions
- Tissue hypoxia
- Malnutrition
- Physical: altered mobility
- Psychological: orientation

External
- Chemical
  - Drugs (abuse or withdrawal)
  - Alcohol (abuse or withdrawal)
  - Other substances, such as glue, fabric softener aerosol (abuse or withdrawal)

Patient Outcomes

The child will

- agree to abstain from using substance or to participate in substance abuse treatment program.
- remain safe and without injury.

Nursing Interventions	Rationales
Assess for personal or environmental risk factors. Complete drug history, including substances used, duration and frequency of use of each substance, when last used, typical amount of usage, and source (if possible).	Knowledge of usage patterns is essential for planning care.
Assess for evidence of disorientation, flashbacks, hallucinations, seizures, delirium, and psychomotor agitation.	Evidence of these problems indicates a need for special safety requirements.
Use laboratory testing of blood and urine to validate history given by child.	Subjective history may be inadequate.
Assess current emotional state, particularly for evidence of depression, suicidal tendencies, or increased aggression that might lead to violence.	Significant changes in emotional state can result from the substances themselves or during withdrawal.
Assess child and family's knowledge about substance abuse.	
Develop a plan with child and family to maintain child's safety. If safety cannot be ensured at home, consider the need for hospitalization.	The child's safety must be the first priority.
Monitor child's progress for evidence of termination of substance abuse.	Relapses are quite common.
Teach child and family members about the effects of substances used on the body. Emphasize that a positive prognosis depends on abstinence.	Many patients lack accurate information about the effects of substances on the body.

▼

NURSING DIAGNOSIS: INEFFECTIVE INDIVIDUAL COPING

Related To
- Inadequate support systems
- Unrealistic perceptions
- Inadequate coping method
- Strong peer pressure
- Dysfunctional family system
- Possible genetic component
- Inadequately developed ego

Defining Characteristics

Inability to meet role expectations
Inability to problem solve
Alteration in societal participation
Destructive behavior toward self or others
Verbal manipulation
High accident rate
Excessive smoking
Excessive drinking/alcohol proneness
Overuse of prescribed tranquilizers
Poor self-esteem
Emotional tension
Chronic depression
Low frustration tolerance
Inability to delay gratification
Denial of problems

Patient Outcomes

- The child will utilize adaptive coping skills instead of substance abuse to deal with life stresses.
- The child and family will acknowledge child's substance abuse problem.

Nursing Interventions	Rationales
Assess social skills, communication skills, assertiveness skills, problem-solving skills, and ability to express emotions appropriately.	Child may be lacking sufficient coping skills in all or any of these areas.

Nursing Interventions	**Rationales**
Confront the child and/or family about denial of the seriousness of the substance abuse problem. Confrontation should be based on caring, with the purpose of limiting fantasizing about the abusing lifestyle and helping the child or family members recognize the problems created by the substance abuse.	The child and his/her family must be able to recognize the use of the substance as a significant problem.
Limit manipulative behaviors consistently in interactions. Establish reasonable consequences for unacceptable behaviors. Work with family to develop a plan for dealing with inappropriate behaviors.	Child has demonstrated inability to maintain reasonable limits; consistent implementation of limits helps teach this to the child, promoting ego development.
Encourage verbalization of feelings.	An impairment of affective expression is common in substance abusers.
Work with the family to help the child learn missing skills, such as assertiveness or problem solving. Provide practice sessions on the needed skills.	Many coping skills can be taught directly. Actual practicing of the skills increases the effectiveness of the learning.
Teach child and family about appropriate support groups, such as Alcoholics Anonymous and Narcotics Anonymous, and the importance of participating in these groups weekly or more often.	Participation in these groups greatly enhances abstinence from the use of substances. They also provide a support system for the child, who often lacks support.
Explore with the child and family members expectations of self and others. Correct distortions of social reality.	
Support the child's ability to be responsible for self at an age-appropriate level, including decision making and problem solving. Point out the constant choices the child has and the positive and negative consequences of available choices.	Age-appropriate independence strengthens the child's sense of self-esteem and enhances ego development, both of which are essential for withstanding negative peer pressure.

▼

NURSING DIAGNOSIS: SELF-ESTEEM DISTURBANCE

Related To
- Dysfunctional family system
- Lack of positive reinforcement
- Impaired ego development
- Feelings of inadequacy

Defining Characteristics

Evaluates self as unable to deal with events

Frequently lacks success in school or other life events

Rationalizes away/rejects positive feedback and exaggerates negative feedback about self

Denial of problems obvious to others

Projection of blame/responsibility for problems

Rationalizes personal failures

Hypersensitivity to criticism

Grandiosity

Self destructive behavior of substance abuse

Impaired interpersonal relationships

Patient Outcomes

The child will
- verbalize desire to remain substance free.
- take steps to begin substance abuse treatment as evidence of increased feelings of self-worth.

Nursing Interventions	Rationales
Identify child's perceptions about self, including strengths and limitations.	
Assess family's feelings toward the child and their willingness to work together as a family to resolve the problems.	The family members may have ambivalent feelings toward the child that may interfere with their ability to engage in treatment.
Provide opportunities for the child to experience successes with new activities by starting with the simple and moving to the more complex.	Success with new activities contributes to self-esteem.

Nursing Interventions	Rationales
Encourage the child to participate with peers in substance abuse treatment program where he/she will receive positive feedback as well as appropriate confrontation.	Participation will help the child feel less isolated and alone.
Teach the child assertiveness, effective communication, and problem-solving skills.	Improved ability to interact effectively and get reasonable needs met enhances self-esteem.
Teach the family to recognize the influence of their communication styles on the child.	Negative interactional patterns may exist that contribute to the child's difficulties with self-esteem.
Assess the child's functioning in school (age appropriate).	
Contact the school system and develop a plan for meeting the child's needs during school time.	School is an important place for obtaining recognition and experiencing success that can improve self-esteem.
Provide positive reinforcement for accomplishments, even if apparently small, as well as affirmations for being.	The child needs both for the development of self-esteem.

▼

DISCHARGE PLANNING/CONTINUITY OF CARE

Refer child and family
- for substance abuse treatment and/or psychiatric care. (Without specialized treatment, substance abuse is very difficult to stop. Family involvement is very important in achieving resolution of the substance abuse.)
- to dietitian for meal planning.
- to Alcoholics Anonymous, Narcotics Anonymous, or other substance abuse support groups for children or adolescents. Encourage consistent, active participation by the youth and the family.

$\mathcal{S}$YPHILIS

Jeffrey Zurlinden, RN, MS

$\mathbf{S}$yphilis is a sexually transmitted disease (STD). The incidence of syphilis in sexually active adolescents has risen in recent years. Infection in a young child may indicate sexual abuse. If untreated, syphilis progresses over the remainder of the patient's lifetime through four stages: primary, secondary, latent, and tertiary. Screening blood tests are vital to detect syphilis; however, patients who are concurrently infected with human immunodeficiency virus (HIV) may remain falsely negative for syphilis serologies. This care plan does not describe the care of a patient with tertiary syphilis or a newborn with congenital syphilis.

ETIOLOGY

Bacterial infection with *Treponema pallidum*

CLINICAL MANIFESTATIONS

- Primary syphilis: chancre
- Secondary syphilis: nonpruritic skin rash
- Latent syphilis: asymptomatic period; may last decades
- Tertiary syphilis: degenerative changes in heart, central nervous system, and skeletal system, including paresis, dementia, aortic insufficiency, and tabes dorsalis

CLINICAL/DIAGNOSTIC FINDINGS

Positive syphilis serology

▼

NURSING DIAGNOSIS: INFECTION

Related To presence of infectious organisms

Defining Characteristics

History of sexual contact with an infected person
Positive syphilis serology
Presence of chancre, condylomata lata, or rash

Patient Outcomes

Patient will exhibit no signs of infection, as evidenced by declining syphilis serology titers.

Nursing Interventions	Rationales
Check local and state regulations to determine if STDs in minors are reportable to the Health Department.	
Determine date of last sexual contact, number of sexual partners, and description of recent sexual activities.	This provides information regarding behaviors that increases risk of STDs.
Assess syphilis serology results.	Low-titer biological false-positive results are possible during pregnancy, autoimmune disease, or other infections. Confirmatory test will exclude biological false-positive result in patients without previous syphilis infection. Because infected person has a negative syphilis serology for the first 4–6 weeks after infection, contacts of infected people are treated as if they are infected.
Inspect skin, mouth, vagina, rectum, penis, and perineum for chancre, condylomata lata, and rashes.	
Obtain history of previous STDs.	
Screen for other STDs, hepatitis B, and HIV.	Patients with one STD are at a higher risk for a concomitant STD.
In women, obtain menstrual history, including date of last period.	

Nursing Interventions	Rationales
Determine method of and compliance with birth control.	Contracting STDs suggests no use/improper use of condoms. Adolescents are especially high risk for pregnancy. Nurse should use this opportunity for health screening/education.
Check local and state regulations to determine if minors can receive abortion or birth control counseling without parental notification or consent.	
Perform pregnancy test.	This is necessary for early detection of pregnancy. Some women may become pregnant before they begin menstruating. Some drugs have a teratogenic effect. Fetal transmission and the development of congenital syphilis depends on the stage of the mother's infection. Fetal damage can be prevented if disease is treated before the 16th week of gestation.
Check local and state regulations to determine if minors can receive treatment for STDs transmitted diseases without parental notification or consent.	
Administer antibiotics as ordered.	Treatment changes in response to the development of new antibiotics. Usually intramuscular (IM) penicillin G is given; however, the dose and length of treatment depend on the stage of syphilis. Follow the current guidelines from the Centers for Disease Control (CDC) or local Health Department.
Observe for possible anaphylactic reaction to IM antibiotics given during clinic visit.	

Nursing Interventions	Rationales
Dispense condoms.	The use of latex condoms is the most effective means of preventing the spread of disease during sexual contact.
Instruct patient to inform all recent sexual partners of possible exposure to syphilis and need for treatment.	Untreated asymptomatic sexual partners are common source of reinfection.
Determine if sexual contact was consensual. Refer to social service if abuse is suspected.	

▼

NURSING DIAGNOSIS: KNOWLEDGE DEFICIT

Related To new diagnosis

Defining Characteristics
Patient asks many questions
Patient asks few questions
Patient has history of repeated infections
Patient is unable to state the causes, treatment, and prevention of syphilis

Patient Outcomes
Patient will state
- medication schedule and side effects.
- date of return visits.
- how to use condoms to prevent future infections.

Nursing Interventions	Rationales
Assess patient's present level of understanding.	Misconceptions can increase anxiety/fear and foster spread of STD.
Instruct about medication schedule and side effects of antibiotics.	Course of treatment depends on the stage of syphilis. Follow the current guidelines from the CDC or local Health Department.
Instruct to refrain from vaginal, rectal, and pharyngeal sexual intercourse until patient and partners have completed treatment.	

Nursing Interventions	Rationales
Instruct on mode of transmission: from chancre site to portion of patient's body that touches chancre. Chancres may be hidden in vagina, rectum, or mouth.	
Instruct patient to use latex condoms or use other nonintercourse sexual methods to prevent future infections.	Latex condoms are an effective barrier against contact with chancres.
Inform patient of signs and symptoms of Jarish-Herxheimer reaction (fever, chills, malaise, myalgia, and sore throat 6–8 hr after antibiotic therapy; subsiding after 12–24 hr). Patients may need aspirin for symptomatic relief.	Occurs in 50% of patients with primary syphilis and 75% of those with secondary syphilis.

NURSING DIAGNOSIS: INEFFECTIVE MANAGEMENT OF THERAPEUTIC REGIMEN

Related To
- Unwillingness to comply with treatment, prevention, or informing sexual partners
- Complexity of treatment regimen

Defining Characteristics
Titer of syphilis serology that does not decrease after treatment
Missed return visits
Incorrect pill count at return visit
Inadequate blood level of antibiotic

Patient Outcomes
Patient will
- complete course of treatment.
- notify sexual partners.
- keep return visits for follow-up serology.
- use condoms to prevent infection.

Nursing Interventions	Rationales
Compare actual effect and expected therapeutic effect.	

Nursing Interventions	Rationales
Plot patient's pattern of returning for tests of cure or follow-up visits.	
Determine social support systems and presence of significant others.	Interpersonal influence can impact on compliance with treatment regimen.
Assess patient's and significant other's beliefs about current illness and treatment plan.	How one perceives susceptibility, severity, and threat of disease impacts on health behaviors.
Assess quality of relationship between patient and health care workers and health care facility.	
Role play to practice informing sexual partners of possible exposure to syphilis.	This gives patient an opportunity to rehearse situations and allows nurse to provide feedback.
Suggest IM medications or short-term therapy if patient has a history of not taking oral medication.	IM medication eliminates the patient's need to participate in treatment.
Role play to practice new behaviors in situations leading to reinfection (such as saying "no" or using condoms).	
Develop a positive relationship with the patient that encourages participation in treatment decisions.	The nurse-patient relationship is based on recognition of patient's right to self-determination and capacity for self-management, with focus on decision making and goal attainment.
Determine with the patient the plan of treatment he/she is most likely to complete.	Involving the patient in planning the regimen improves compliance.

NURSING DIAGNOSIS: ALTERED SEXUALITY PATTERNS

Related To
- Imposed restrictions
- Fear
- Risk of contagion

Defining Characteristics

Patient or significant other expresses concern about the effects syphilis and treatment have on their expressions of physical intimacy.

Patient Outcome

Patient will state ways of expressing physical intimacy during treatment.

Nursing Interventions	Rationales
Determine patient's or significant other's concerns.	
Determine if concerns also are related to fears about acquired immunodeficiency syndrome (AIDS).	An STD diagnosis may provoke fear of AIDS that alters sexual behavior.
Assess perception of meaning of syphilis infection.	This provides opportunity to correct misconceptions.
Elicit patient's feeling about limits on sexual behavior.	
Explore ways to express physical intimacy during treatment excluding vaginal, rectal, and pharyngeal intercourse.	Restrictions on sexual activity should not deprive the couple of other activities that convey the message that they are loved and desired.
Explore ways to express physical intimacy that do not lead to reinfection.	Barrier contraception with latex condoms is effective.

▼

DISCHARGE PLANNING/CONTINUITY OF CARE

- Arrange gynecology consult.
- Schedule patient to return for repeat serology tests (usually performed at 1, 6, 12, and 24 months after therapy).
- Instruct patient to return sooner for routine screening if high-risk sexual behavior continues.
- Refer for HIV counseling and testing. (Syphilis may be more difficult to detect and progress more rapidly in HIV-infected women).
- Refer to
  - family planning clinic
  - support group.

UNDESCENDED TESTICLE (CRYPTORCHIDISM)

Nedra Skale, RN, MS, CNA

An undescended testis, or cryptorchidism, refers to a testis that is not in the scrotum. It is to be distinguished from a retractile testis, which tends to stay in the inguinal canal but can be brought down into the scrotum by gentle manipulation. An ectopic testis is one that has strayed from the inguinal canal into the thigh or perineum.

ETIOLOGIES

- Prematurity
- Heredity

CLINICAL MANIFESTATIONS

On physical exam, the testicle or testicles cannot be palpated in the scrotum.

CLINICAL/DIAGNOSTIC FINDINGS

None

▼

NURSING DIAGNOSIS: HIGH RISK FOR INJURY

Risk Factors
- Prematurity
- Undescended testicle at birth
- History of scrotal pain/swelling

Patient Outcomes

- The child's testicles will remain in scrotum.
- Risk of infertility and hormonal dysfunction will be reduced.

Nursing Interventions	Rationales
Assess child's history for 1. prematurity	The testes descend into the scrotal sac during the last trimester of pregnancy.
2. undescended testicle at birth	
3. incidence of scrotal pain/ swelling	This may indicate a torsion and possibly subsequent atrophy of testis.
With warm hands, palpate the scrotal sac; if the testes are not descended, palpate the inguinal canal on the involved side.	The testes are sensitive to cold and touch and will retract reflexively (cremasteric reflex).
Determine if testes in the canal can be descended with gentle, intermittent pressure.	The testes that can be descended during infancy may descend permanently on its own. The testes that cannot be descended, especially past 1 year of age, requires surgical intervention (orchiopexy).
Explain the need for regular, consistent follow-up if surgery is delayed to see if testicle will descend spontaneously.	Lack of follow-up can result in permanent testicular damage.
Explain hormonal therapy if ordered. 1. hCG therapy involves intramuscular injections three times a week for 10 doses. 2. Side effects include penile growth and frequent erections during therapy. 3. Descent should occur within 1 week after completion of injections if successful (10–30% success rate).	If the testes is low lying in the inguinal canal, descent sometimes occurs following injections of human chorionic gonadotropin (hCG).

Nursing Interventions	Rationales
Reinforce the need for surgery in the following cases: 1. bilateral undescended testicles 2. bilateral undescended testis by age 3 years	Surgery is necessary because 1. body heat damages testes, causing sterility 2. the testes produce testosterone necessary for pubertal development 3. descent improves size and shape of scrotum
3. dysplastic testes or those high in the abdomen require orchiectomy.	Risk of neoplastic changes increases if left untreated.

▼

NURSING DIAGNOSIS: BODY IMAGE DISTURBANCE (PARENT/CHILD)

Related To biophysical dysfunction

Defining Characteristics
Absent body part
Refusal to touch or look at body part
Withdrawal from social contacts
Self-destructive behavior
Unwillingness to discuss the defect

Patient Outcomes
- The child will participate in school and social activities.
- The child/parent will be able to discuss condition and treatment choices.
- The child's physical appearance will improve.

Nursing Interventions	Rationales
Assess child's and parents' reaction to diagnosis.	
Assess older child's experience with peers and feelings about problem.	A school-age child is especially conscious of his body and reacts to being different from peers. The child may have experienced the ridicule of peers.

Nursing Interventions	Rationales
Explain to the parents the psychological impact of an undescended testicle on the child, as well as the long-term potential for infertility and hormonal dysfunction.	Surgery performed before age 3 years will alleviate body image concerns.
Explain that, if testes are dysplastic/atrophied, an orchiectomy may be done and a prosthetic replacement can be performed when the child is older.	A prosthesis will make the young man appear normal. Fertility will be impaired.

▼

DISCHARGE PLANNING/CONTINUITY OF CARE

- Frequent follow-up is necessary during infancy to evaluate testicular position.
- Instruct parents to return immediately if symptoms of torsion exist.
- Refer to pediatric surgeon, urologist, and/or endocrinologist.

URINARY TRACT INFECTION

Peggy Cowling, RNC, MSN

An invasion of bacteria in any part of the urinary tract, which includes the bladder (cystitis), the urethra (urethritis), and the kidneys (pyelonephritis), is called urinary tract infection (UTI). UTIs in children more readily lead to pyelonephritis and renal deterioration than do those in adults.

ETIOLOGIES

- Short female urethra in close proximity to vagina and anus
- Incomplete emptying and overdistention of bladder
- Concentrated, alkaline urine

CLINICAL MANIFESTATIONS

See Nursing Diagnosis: Infection, Defining Characteristics

CLINICAL/DIAGNOSTIC FINDINGS

Positive urine culture

▼

NURSING DIAGNOSIS: INFECTION

Related To bacteria in the urinary tract:
- *Escherichia coli*
- *Enterobacteriaceae*
- *Klebsiella*
- *Proteus*
- *Pseudomonas*

Defining Characteristics

Neonate
Asymptomatic
Nonspecific
Vomiting
Diarrhea
Temperature
Instability
Lethargy
Poor feeding
Poor weight gain
Irritable
Malodorous urine
Diaper rash

Toddler
High fever
Abdominal pain
Malodorous urine
Weak stream
Dribbling
Urgency/frequency
Pain/burning
Inflammed urethra

Older Child
Fever
Chills
Dysuria
Frequency
Enuresis
Abdominal pain
Flank pain
Anorexia

Patient Outcomes

The child will display no signs of infection, as evidenced by a normal temperature, and no irritability, anorexia, diarrhea, or dysuria.

Nursing Interventions	Rationales
Inspect diaper area every half hour until void is observed.	Increases chance of observing stream of urine for abnormalities in an infant or toddler.

Nursing Interventions	Rationales
Inspect general area for inflammation, diaper rash, and pinworms.	This may identify local area of inflammation that contributes to diagnosis of UTI, which can have nonspecific symptoms in infants and toddlers.
Obtain health history from parents/child regarding behavior changes, unexplained fever/abdominal pain, and change in voiding pattern.	Symptomatology guides diagnosis.
Collect midstream clean-catch urine specimen or assist with suprapubic aspiration or catheterization.	Only a urine culture can properly diagnose a UTI; urine specimen easily can be contaminated with perineal bacteria.
Assess temperature.	Because UTIs can be very nonspecific, unexplained fevers should be evaluated for UTI.
Encourage increased fluid intake; try acidic juices like orange/cranberry.	This dilutes the urine and may reduce the fever. Acidic urine is less hospitable to bacteria.
Teach parents proper administration of antibiotics, including dose, time, route, amount, name of drug, and purpose (usually amoxicillin or Gantrisin).	Adherence to prescribed regimen is essential for optimum results. Entire course of drug must be completed to prevent recurrence.
Teach strategies to prevent occurrence of infection: 1. avoid bubble baths 2. avoid tight fitting clothes, diapers 3. perform "front-to-back" perineal hygiene 4. encourage fluids 5. avoid "holding" urine 6. avoid constipation 7. urinate after sexual intercourse (if adolescent is sexually active)	Constipation obstructs neck of bladder in young children, leading to residual urine.
Instruct parents to check routinely for infection.	Repeat UTIs can lead to pyelonephritis and renal deterioration.

Nursing Interventions	Rationales
Instruct older child/adolescent to report signs of infection as soon as noticed.	Early diagnosis and treatment can prevent tissue destruction and severe pain.

▼

NURSING DIAGNOSIS: PAIN

Related To inflammation of urinary tract

Defining Characteristics
Irritability
Poor feeding
Crying on urination
Hesitancy to urinate
Abdominal complaints
Flank tenderness
Complaints of pain

Patient Outcomes
- The child will
  - be able to urinate without burning or pain.
  - have no complaint of abdominal or flank pain.
- The infant will
  - not be irritable.
  - feed well.
  - not cry on urination.

Nursing Interventions	Rationales
Tailor assessment to child's age and developmental level.	Children often cannot report pain because of limited verbal skills.
Learn what words child uses for pain.	This ensures more accurate assessment by respecting families' preferences and avoids confusion.
Use behavioral observation when language barriers exist, such as physiological measure (heart rate and blood pressure), vocalizations, body posture, and activity.	
Obtain parents' report of child's pain.	Parents know children best and will identify personality changes more readily than health care workers.

Nursing Interventions	Rationales
Provide swaddling, rocking, and pacifiers for infants undergoing procedures or who are irritable.	This provides sensorimotor input to distract from discomfort.
Encourage rest and application of heat for abdominal/flank pain.	This promotes muscular relaxation, which decreases pain perception.
Provide older children distraction techniques and play therapy.	
Give acetaminophen to control fever and pain.	
Encourage increased fluid intake.	Increased fluid intake will increase urine output, diluting urine and increasing comfort with voids.
Prepare child and family for additional testing to rule out anatomical problems.	An intravenous pyelogram or voiding cystourethrogram may be ordered in the event of repeat infections in a very young child.

▼

DISCHARGE PLANNING/CONTINUITY OF CARE

- Follow up in 2 days; send repeat urine culture.
- Instruct on necessity of repeat urine culture after antibiotics are completed. If urine cannot be collected in office, give instructions on urine collection at home. Provide collection device and/or cup. Specimen should be refrigerated until brought to office or lab.
- Provide referral for urological evaluation.

REFERENCES: COMMON CHILDHOOD DISORDERS

Berman, S. (1991). *Pediatric decision making*. Philadelphia, PA: B. C. Decker.

Buckley, H. (1992). Syphilis: A review and update of this "new" infection of the '90s. *Nurse Practitioner, 17*(8), 25–32.

Cates, W. & Tooney, K. E. (1990). Sexually transmitted diseases: Overview of the situation. *Primary Care, 17*(1), 1–27.

Cervisi, J., Chapman, M., Niklas, B., & Tamaoka, C. (1991). Office management of the infant with colic. *Journal of Pediatric Health Care, 5*(4) 184–190.

Dawkins, B. J. (1990). Genital herpes simplex infections. *Primary Care, 17*(1), 95–113.

Della Bella, L. (1992). Steroidophobia and the pulmonary patient, *American Journal of Nursing, 92*(2), 26–29.

Diacon, N. V. (1992). Nursing interventions for children with attention-deficit hyperactivity disorder. *Bulletin of the Menniger Clinic, 56*(3), 313–320.

Engle, N. S. (1990). Phenobarbital for pediatric febrile seizures: Risk-benefit update. *American Journal of Maternal Child Nursing 15*(4), 257.

Erhardt, D. & Baker, B. (1990). The effects of behavioral parent training on families with young hyperactive children. *Journal of Behavioral Therapy, 21*(2), 121–132.

Finelli, L. (1991). Evaluation of the child with acute abdominal pain. *Journal of Pediatric Health Care, 5*(5), 251–256.

Graham, J. M. & Blanco, J. D. (1990). Chlamydial infections. *Primary Care, 17*(1), 85–93.

Gulanick, M., Puzas, M., & Wilson, C. (1992). *Nursing care plans for newborn and children: Acute and critical care*, St. Louis, MO: Mosby-Year Book.

Handsfield, H. H. (1991). Recent developments in STDs: I. Bacterial diseases. *Hospital Practice, 26*(7), 47–56.

Handsfield, H. H. (1991). Recent developments in STDs: II. Viral and other syndromes. *Hospital Practice, 27*(1), 175–200.

Handsfield, H. H. & Hammerschlag, M. (1992). Chlamydia: A diagnostic challenge. *Patient Care, 26*, 69–84.

Holaday, B. (1991). The care of children with minimal brain dysfunction: A Roy adaptation analysis. *Journal of Pediatric Nursing, 6*, 290–292.

Hyman, H., Tildesley, E., Lichtenstein, E., Ary, D., & Sherman, L. (1990). Parent-adolescent problem-solving interactions and drug use. *American Journal of Drug and Alcohol Abuse, 16*(3/4), 239–258.

Jenny, C. (1992). Sexually transmitted diseases and child abuse. *Pediatric Annals, 21*(8), 497–503.

Keefe, M. & Froese-Fretz, A. (1991). Living with an irritable infant: Maternal perspectives. *The American Journal of Maternal/Child Nursing, 16*(5), 255–259.

Keller, M. L., Jadack, R. A., & Mims, K. F. (1991). Perceived stressors and coping responses in persons with recurrent genital herpes. *Research in Nursing and Health*, 14(6), 421–430.

Kelly, D. P. & Aylward, G. P. (1992). Attention deficits in school-aged children and adolescents: Current issues and practices. *Pediatric Clinics of North America*, 39(3), 487–512.

Kenner, C. & Lott, J. (1990). Parent transition after discharge from the NICU. *Neonatal Network*, 9(2), 31–37.

Kranzler, E., Schaffer, D., Wasserman, G., & Davies, E. (1990). Early childhood bereavement. *Journal of the American Academy of Child and Adolescent Psychiatry*, 29(4), 513–520.

LaGreca, A., Follansbee, D., & Skyler, J. S. (1990). Developmental and behavioral aspects of diabetes management in youngsters. *CHC*, 19(3), 132–139.

Libbus, M. K. (1992). Condoms as primary prevention in sexually active women. *The American Journal of Maternal/Child Nursing*, 17(5), 256–260.

Lindell, K. O. & Mazzocco, M. C. (1990). Breaking bronchospasm's grip with MDI's. *American Journal of Nursing* 90(3), 34–39.

Moy, J. B. & Clasen, M. E. (1990). The patient with gonococcal infection. *Primary Care*, 17(1), 59–83.

Nettina, S. L. & Kaufman, F. H. (1990). Diagnosis and management of sexually transmitted genital lesions. *Nurse Practitioner*, 15(1), 20–39.

Newcomer, S. & Baldwin, W. (1992). Demographics of adolescent sexual behavior, contraception, and STDs. *Journal of School Health*, 62(7), 265–270.

Noble, R. C. (1990). Sequelae of sexually transmitted diseases. *Primary Care*, 17(1), 173–182.

Norris-Berkemeyer, S. (1991). Childhood lead poisoning. *CHART*, 88(8), 5–6.

Opie, N. D. (1992). Childhood and adolescent bereavement. *Annual Review of Nursing Research*, 10, 127–141.

Opie, N. D., Goodwin, T., Finke, L., Beattey, J. M., Lee, B., & Van Epps, J. (1992). The effect of a bereavement group experience on bereaved children's and adolescents' affective and somatic distress. *Journal of Child and Adolescent Psychiatric and Mental Health Nursing*, 5(1), 20–26.

Perry, C. L. & Kelder, S. H. (1992). Models for effective prevention. *Journal of Adolescent Health*, 13(5), 355–363.

Pisterman, S., Firestone, P., McGrath, P., Goodman, J. T., Webster, I., Mallory, R., & Goffin, B. (1992). The role of parent training in the treatment of preschoolers with ADDH. *American Journal of Orthopsychiatry*, 62(3), 397–408.

Raffensperger, J. G. (1990). *Swenson's pediatric surgery*. Norwalk, CT: Appleton & Lange.

Rakel, R. (1990). *Textbook of family practice*. Philadelphia, PA: W. B. Saunders.

Reinke, L. F. & Hoffman, L. A., (1992). How to teach asthma co-management. *American Journal of Nursing, 92*(10), 40–46.

Reynolds, S. L. & Jaffe, D. M. (1990). Quick triage of children with abdominal pain. *Emergency Medicine, 22*(14), 39–42.

Shaw, N. (1990). Common surgical problems in the newborn. *Journal of Perinatal & Neonatal Nursing, 3*(3), 50–65.

Skale, N. (1992) *Manual of pediatric nursing procedures*. Philadelphia, PA: J. B. Lippincott Co.

Tarter, R. (1990). Evaluation and treatment of adolescent substance abuse: A decision tree method. *American Journal of Drug and Alcohol Abuse, 16*(1/2), 1–46.

Tillman, J. (1992). Syphilis: An old disease, a contemporary perinatal problem. *Journal of Obstetric, Gynecologic, and Neonatal Nursing, 21*(3), 209–213.

Tucker, J. A., Vuchinich, R. E., & Gladsjo, J. A. (1990–1991). Environmental influences on relapse in substance disorders. *International Journal of Addictions, 25*(7A-8A), 1017–1050.

Washburn, P. (1991). Identification, assessment, and referral of adolescent drug abusers. *Pediatric Nursing, 17*(2), 137–140, 142–143.

Zambelli, G. C. & DeRosa, A. P. (1992). Bereavement support groups for school-aged children: Theory, intervention, and case example. *American Journal of Orthopsychiatry, 62*(4), 484–493.

Health Teaching Guides

▼

CAST CARE

Michele Knoll Puzas, RNC, MHPE

Children's injuries involving fractures occur frequently as a result of motor vehicle accidents and play and sports injuries. Casts are used to immobilize the fracture and permit healing in correct alignment.

1. Discuss type of cast and its purpose with parent and child.
2. Instruct child/family to handle new cast gently and allow to dry thoroughly. A plaster cast may take a day or longer to dry depending on its size. A Fiberglas cast dries more quickly, in 8–10 hr. Provide sling to upper extremity if indicated. Encourage elevation of affected limb.
3. Instruct child/family to keep the padding/stockinette/cast dry.
4. Instruct child and family to observe for and report immediately
   - increased swelling
   - increased pain
   - pallor, tingling, or lack of feeling
   - bleeding or other discharge through cast
   - foul odor from cast
5. Discuss assistance child will need with activities of daily living specific to limb(s) casted and to child's age and developmental level. Assistance may be required for
   - bathing
   - ambulation
   - repositioning
   - feeding
   - toileting
6. Instruct the child/family not to put anything down the cast. Encourage the use of diversions to keep child's thoughts away from cast/itching. An oral medication may be considered if itching is severe.
7. Request parent to return to office or call if cast has become very loose, cracked, soft, or very wet.
8. Make sure parent knows when to return for cast removal. Casts should never be removed at home.

$\mathcal{C}$IRCUMCISION CARE

Caroline Reich, RN, MS

Circumcision is the removal of the foreskin of the penis. In the past, the procedure was routinely performed on newborns and is still a common sociocultural and religious choice. The procedure also may be performed for medical reasons, such as phimosis.

1. Teach parents care of the circumcised penis:
   - Keep the glans of the penis covered with a lubricated gauze dressing the first 24 hr after the procedure.
   - Once the dressing has been removed, apply a small amount of Bacitracin, A & D, or petroleum jelly directly to the glans for several days after the procedure. Lubricant protects the fresh circumcision site from adhering to the diaper and from direct contact with urine or feces.

NOTE: Lubricant is *not* needed in an infant who had a bell circumcision. No special dressing is required.

   - Cleanse the penis with clear water only during the first few days after the gauze is removed. Soap may be irritating.
   - Wait until after the circumcision site has healed before manipulating the foreskin remnants in an attempt to prevent adhesions. Forcibly attempting to "loosen" the remnants of the foreskin can cause bleeding of the freshly circumcised penis.

2. Instruct parents to check with their health care provider to ascertain whether any additional measures are needed to prevent adhesions from developing. This is dependent on the technique of the physician who performed the circumcision. Individual practice may vary as to how much foreskin remains after the procedure.

3. Teach parents the characteristics of the healing process, and signs and symptoms of infection and other complications:
   - Instruct parents that any bleeding, lack of or difficulty voiding, odor, or discharge should be reported to the physician.
   - Instruct parents that a yellowish, adherent exudate (which is part of the granulation process) may appear on the penis and should not be removed. This exudate is a normal part of the healing process.

4. Teach parents comfort measures that can be employed for several days after the procedure, such as:
   - Applying the diaper loosely and positioning the infant on his side. This will prevent undue pressure against the penis and will make the infant more comfortable.
   - Using cloth diapers instead of disposable diapers. Some practitioners believe that cloth diapers are less irritating to the circumcision site than disposables.

DENTAL HYGIENE: CARIES PREVENTION

Marlene Smith RNC, MSN, FNP

Dental hygiene and the prevention of caries is best accomplished when good habits are begun in infancy. The child who becomes accustomed to dental care is more likely to be compliant later in childhood.

1. Review with parents the common causes for dental caries:
   - infant's/child's feeding habits
   - lack of adequate oral hygiene habits
   - residential water of less than 0.7 ppm of fluoride concentration
2. Explain the development of dental caries:
   - begins with plaque formation on teeth; results from interaction of bacteria (usually *Streptococcus mutans*), diet, and tooth susceptibility.
   - results in localized, gradually progressive decay and disintegration of the tooth dentin (begun by acid breakup of the enamel tooth surface).

For infants/toddlers
3. Assess behaviors that increase risk of caries:
   - bottle propping
   - prolonged bottle or breast feeding
   - falling asleep during feeding
   - being put to sleep with carbohydrate liquids in a bottle

NOTE: Refined carbohydrates have been clearly shown to have cariogenic potential. Pooling and stasis of liquid occurs in a sleeping child's mouth.

4. Instruct parents to use fluoride supplementation if an infant is exclusively breast-fed.
5. Assess for fluoride supplementation in formula prepared for infant. Use if water supply contains less than 0.7 ppm of fluoride.

For older child
6. Inform parents of the ages for the greatest carie activity: 4–8 years and 12–18 years.
7. Assess child's oral hygiene habits.
8. Provide instruction on proper oral hygiene:
   - tooth brushing
     - after each meal, especially after foods of high sugar content

- should both remove food debris and stimulate gingivae
- using fluoridated toothpaste. Explain that fluoride has been found to prevent dental caries by both systemic and topical routes. The exact method is not known. Hypotheses include:
  - Fluoride makes enamel less soluble by changing its crystalline structure.
  - By using fluoride, cariogenic bacteria in plaque is lessened.
  - With fluoride present, bacterial adhesion is inhibited on the enamel surface.
- rinsing (not swallowing) with antiplaque rinse (rinses can be toxic in large amounts)
- flossing
  - important for removing plaque and food debris *between* permanent teeth
  - should be performed daily by child or parent (baby teeth are not in close enough contact to require flossing between teeth)
9. Provide opportunity for child to review diagrams of teeth, and to practice brushing/flossing while in the clinic setting.
10. Instruct parents to use supplemental fluoride from birth to age 13 if residential water supply contains less than 0.7 ppm of fluoride.
11. Explain importance of regular dental exams and fluoride treatments as needed.
12. Instruct child to avoid between meals sweets and to eat a balanced nutritious diet.
13. *For all ages,* refer to dentist, pedodontist, orthodontist, or oral surgeon if indicated.

$\mathcal{J}$MMUNIZATIONS

Michele Knoll Puzas, RNC, MHPE

Immunizations and their effects on the child are topics of concern for parents. The importance of immunizations and the diseases they prevent must be explained.

1. Explain to parents the importance of immunizations and disease prevention. See Table 55.1.
2. Give parent printed material explaining immunizations: U.S. Department of Health, Centers for Disease Control, or American Academy of Pediatrics guidelines.
3. Explain the immunization schedule. See Tables 55.2 and 55.3.
4. Inform parents of potential side effects of immunizations:
   - expected effects
     - irritability
     - low-grade fever (< 102°F)
     - redness, sensitivity at site
     - mild rash
   - serious effects
     - fever > 104°F
     - inconsolable crying for more than 3 hr
     - unusual high-pitched crying
     - excessive sleepiness
     - difficulty waking up
     - limpness, paleness
     - convulsions
5. Obtain consent if needed.
6. Give parents a record of the child's immunizations. This should be updated at every visit.
7. Instruct parents to give acetaminophen every 4 hr. (Children should not be given aspirin because of the strong association between aspirin use, viral illness, and development of Reye's syndrome.)
8. Instruct parents to call or return to office if serious side effects occur.

Table 55.1 • Childhood Diseases and Their Complications

Disease	Complications
Diphtheria	Epistaxis, toxemia, myocarditis, septic shock, death
Tetanus (lockjaw)	Muscular rigidity, convulsions, asphyxia
Pertussis (whooping cough)	Pneumonia, atelectasis
Polio	Paralysis, respiratory arrest
Measles (rubeola)	Fever, pneumonia, encephalitis
Mumps	Encephalitis, deafness, orchitis with sterility
Rubella	Teratogenic during first trimester
Haemophilus type b influenzae	Pneumonia, encephalitis
Hepatitis	Liver damage, systemic damage, death

▼

Table 55.2 • Suggested Routine Immunization Schedule

Age	Immunization
Birth	HBV
1 month	HBV
2 months	DTP, TOPV
4 months	DTP, TOPV
6 months	DTP, TOPV
12 months	HBV, TB skin test
15 months	MMR
18 months	DTP, TOPV, HiB
4–6 years	DTP, TOPV, (MMR)*
14–16 years	Td (every 10 years)

HBV = hepatitis B vaccine
DTP = diphtheria, tetanus, pertussis vaccine
TOPV = trivalent oral polio vaccine
TB = tuberculin test
HiB = *Haemophilus influenzae* type b vaccine
MMR* = measles, mumps, rubella (*some recommend revaccination)
Td = tetanus and diphtheria toxoid (adult type)

▼

Table 55.3 • Suggested Immunization Schedule for Children Not Immunized in Infancy (> 18 months)

Date	Immunization
First visit	DTP, HBV, TOPV, TB skin test, MMR*
1 month later	HBV
2 months later	DTP, TOPV
4 months later	DTP, HBV, TOPV
≥ 2 years old	HiB
3–4 years old (or preschool)	DTP, TOPV
14–16 years old	Td (then every 10 years)

HBV = hepatitis B vaccine
DTP = diphtheria, tetanus, pertussis vaccine
TOPV = trivalent oral polio vaccine
TB = tuberculin test
MMR* = measles, mumps, rubella (*some recommend revaccination)
HiB = *Haemophilus influenzae* type b vaccine
Td = tetanus and diphtheria toxoid (adult type)

▼

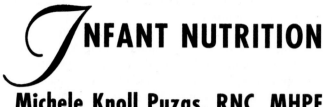

INFANT NUTRITION

Michele Knoll Puzas, RNC, MHPE
Renee Bluml, RD, CNSD

Many new parents have concerns about feeding their infants. Nutrition information should be provided at each routine visit. Discuss the following guidelines:

1. Breast-feeding is the most complete and desirable diet for the infant. Breast-fed babies sometimes gain weight slower than formula-fed infants. This is not a problem and should be explained if mother is concerned.
2. The breast-feeding mother needs to eat a healthy diet for herself and her infant. An iron supplement is needed. Mothers can continue to take iron tablets or prenatal vitamins while breast-feeding.
3. Iron-fortified formula is a complete diet for the infant when prepared correctly as directed.
4. Cow's or evaporated milk should not be started until at least 12 months, and then will require iron supplement or multivitamins with iron.
5. Infants should be held during feeding.
6. Most infants do not require extra water, but it can be offered between feedings, particularly if the weather is hot or overeating is a problem.
7. A fluoride supplement should be considered if the community water is not fluoridated.
8. The amount an infant will eat varies according to age. See Table 56.1.
9. Solid foods should be introduced at 4–6 months, beginning with iron-fortified rice cereal, followed by oatmeal and barley over a span of about 2 weeks. Introduction of new foods at 4–5-day intervals allows for identification of food allergies/intolerances.
10. Use of a small baby spoon for feeding is desirable over placing cereal in bottled formula. Putting solids in the bottle may increase food intake, cause excessive weight gain, and slow baby's development in eating.
11. Introduction of fruits, vegetables, and meats (home puréed or commercially prepared) can begin after cereals have been tolerated. Citrus fruits and juices should be held until at least 6 months of age to de-

crease risk of allergic response. Citrus also acidifies stool, which can irritate the infant's skin.

12. Inform the parent that, as the baby consumes more solid foods, the amount of breast or formula feeding will decline.

13. Finger foods can be introduced at 6–7 months when the infant can sit up and begin to learn to feed himself/herself.

14. Egg yolk can be introduced around 6 months, but egg white should not be offered until the end of the first year because of its association with allergic reaction.

15. At about 8 months, the use of a cup can be introduced to the baby. The infant's motor skills will begin to allow drinking from and holding a cup.

16. Inform parents that, after the first birthday, the child's growth rate slows and so should his/her appetite.

17. See First Year, p 3.

Table 56.1 • Amounts the Average-Size Infant Will Consume

	0–1 Week	1–4 Weeks	1–3 Months	3–6 Months	6–9 Months	10–12 Months
Ounces/ feeding	1–3	2–4	4–6	6–7	7–8	7–8
Feedings/day	6–10	7–8	5–7	4–5	3–4	3
Ave. ounces/ day	16	22	30	32	30	30

NOTE: The parent may notice a sudden increase of feeding frequency at about 6–8 weeks; this is a normal response to growth spurt.

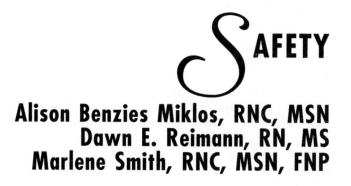

$\mathcal{S}$AFETY

Alison Benzies Miklos, RNC, MSN
Dawn E. Reimann, RN, MS
Marlene Smith, RNC, MSN, FNP

$\mathbf{S}$afety issues should be discussed at each well child visit and related to the child's level of development. Parents need to know what to expect from their child and what preventive measures should be taken.

TRAVEL

- Infants should go home from the hospital in approved car seats. Car seats should be properly installed according to manufacturer's instructions, with regard to child's age and weight.
- Car seats also should be considered for plane travel. Utilize seats labeled and approved for this purpose.
- Seat belts, or approved booster seats with car seat belts, should be used for children over 40 pounds.
- Seat belts should be used every time the child rides in a motor vehicle. Lack of consistency contributes to arguments and risk of injury.

FALLS

- Care should be taken to prevent infant falls from beds and changing tables. Crib side rails should be raised whenever child is unattended.
- As the child grows and becomes more mobile, the crib mattress should be lowered and large toys removed from crib, to prevent the child from climbing out.
- Safety belts in strollers, infant seats, and changing tables should be used. Even with belts, infants should never be left unattended.
- Safety gates should be used to block toddler's access to stairwells or other dangerous areas. Old flexible gates can pinch fingers and potentially harm infants and should be discarded. Infant walkers are not recommended because of the significant relationship between walker use and falls.

CHOKING

- Keep small objects and toys like marbles and beads away from infants and toddlers.
- Avoid balloons, two-piece pacifiers, and any kind of string around a baby's neck that can cause suffocation.
- Keep crib away from cords on window blinds.
- Choose foods carefully when baby begins feeding himself/herself. Items should be small and soft enough for baby to chew.
- Keep baby powder at a safe distance; small infants can suffocate on large amounts of powder. Powders are not recommended because of incidence of inhaling talc into the lungs.

POISON

- Follow directions on medications and vitamins so overdosing does not occur. Measure dose in well-lit room.
- Keep all medicines, soaps, and cleaning solutions up high or locked in cabinets.
- Never refer to medicine as candy.
- Consider types of houseplants available in baby's environment. Many plants are poisonous if consumed and should not be within a baby's reach.
- Never transfer cleaning materials from original containers to cups or bottles; child will assume contents are edible.
- Keep poison control number near telephone.
- Label all poisonous materials (i.e., Mr. Yuk stickers) and explain to child when he/she is able to understand.
- Keep a small bottle of syrup of ipecac on hand, in the event accidental ingestion occurs and vomiting should be induced. Note date of expiration on ipecac.

BURNS

- Make sure smoke alarms are installed in home and batteries are replaced when needed.
- Make sure baby's bath water is not too hot. Never run hot water with baby in tub. Check temperature setting on hot water heater (should be <120°F).
- Keep hot beverages, cooking utensils, and pots and pans out of baby's reach. Always turn handles in away from a toddler's grasp.
- Cover electrical outlets with commercially available plugs and/or place furniture in front of outlets.
- Make sure heating grates and radiators are covered or blocked from baby's access.
- If space heaters must be used, keep a safe distance from baby and use

according to manufacturer's instructions. Do not override safety switches.

SHARP OBJECTS

- Keep all pins, razors, and knives away from baby's reach.
- Select eating utensils safe for young child's use.
- Select safety scissors when child is old enough to use.

DROWNING

- Never leave infants or young children unattended in tub or pool.
- Make sure pools are fenced and locked when not in use and unattended.
- Do not leave fluid-filled buckets in reach of infants or toddlers.
- Keep toilet covers down and bathroom doors locked and/or closed to keep toddlers away from toilet water.
- Do not allow older children/adolescents to swim alone or in unguarded pools/beaches.

$\mathcal{S}$LEEP

Alison Benzies Miklos, RNC, MSN
Dawn E. Reimann, RN, MS

Concerns about sleep patterns are very common during infancy. Careful assessment of an infant's patterns, routines, and behaviors is necessary to determine if a sleep problem exists.

1. Provide parent with information about average sleep patterns:

Table 58.1 • Sleep Patterns of Infants

Age	Sleep Hours/Day	Sleep Hours at Nighttime	Wakeful Periods
Birth–2 months	20	3–4	1–1/ hr
2 months	16–20	6–7	1–2 hr
4 months	15–16	6–8	2 hr
6–8 months	14 (2 naps)	8	4 hr
8–12 months	12 (1 or 2 naps)	8–10	12 hr
18 months	10–12 (1 nap)	8–10	12–14 hr

▼

2. Inform parents that each child develops his/her own sleep pattern based on individual needs.
   • Active infants usually sleep less than calm infants.
   • Breast-fed infants frequently sleep for shorter periods during the night (breast milk is more easily, quickly digested).
   • Newborns do not know the difference between day and night, but usually develop a nocturnal sleep pattern by 3 months.
3. Discuss helpful techniques for establishing appropriate sleep patterns and eliminating sleep problems.
   • Establish consistent bedtime routines (warm bath, rocking, singing, reading a story) to relax infant; helps to accustom infant to nocturnal sleep ritual/pattern.
   • Gradually increase feeding at bedtime.

- From 4 months of age, gradually increase play time during the day and evening hours. Evening play, especially with other family members, will inhibit evening naps, tire infant, and promote night sleep.
- Allow the infant to cry for a few minutes and for gradually longer periods at night so that the infant may learn to self-console and learn that crying does not immediately elicit a parental response.
- Allow/provide consoling techniques (favorite toy and blanket, thumb-sucking, pacifier, open door) to help older infant fall asleep. By 8 months, infants are developing separation anxiety and are sensitive to parent's absence.
- Keep nighttime feeding very subdued (do not turn on lights, play with infant, or unnecessarily change diaper); put infant back to bed immediately after feeding.

4. Inform parents that infant may change sleep patterns as a result of growth spurts, teething pain, and illness. This is a normal occurrence and will resolve.
5. Inform parents of risks involved with allowing infant to sleep in parents' bed, including risk of suffocation and the likelihood that infant will not learn to sleep alone, which may cause problems in the future when parent wants to move child to own bedroom.
6. Inform parents concerned about sudden infant death syndrome (SIDS) that babies at high risk include babies who have
   - low Apgar scores at birth
   - history of apnea requiring resuscitation
   - a sibling death due to SIDS
   - parents who smoke or use drugs
   - low birth weight or premature birth

NOTE: These infants may require home sleep apnea monitoring.

7. For all infants who are not high risk, inform parents of techniques that decrease the risk of SIDS:
   - Place newborns on their side or back. A small towel or blanket is enough to support the infant in a side-lying position.
   - Make sure infant has burped and do not overfeed. Place in bed side-lying if concerned about regurgitation.
   - Make sure sleep surface is flat. Do not place newborns on waterbeds or bean bags or face down on quilts or sheepskin.
8. Explain that risk of SIDS naturally diminishes as the infant grows stronger and is able to change position and turn head.
9. Encourage new mothers to sleep when their infant naps, so they are rested and can enjoy their baby.

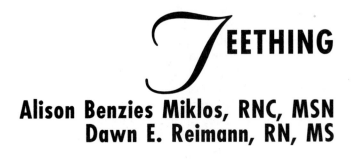

TEETHING

Alison Benzies Miklos, RNC, MSN
Dawn E. Reimann, RN, MS

Teething is a great concern to parents because of the discomfort it causes the infant and the temporary disruption of sleep and feeding patterns. Although a few infants have exhibited low-grade fever and loose stools during a period of teething, these symptoms should be followed for identification of other etiology.

The salivary glands mature at about 3 months of age, so parents may notice an increase in drooling. This is a normal occurrence, and alone does not signal the onset of teething.

1. Inform parents about when their infant may begin teething. Generally the lower incisors erupt first, usually around 6 months, but this can vary. A few infants are born with teeth and some do not teethe until 11–12 months. The later the infant's teeth erupt, the later in childhood they will be lost.

2. Describe symptoms of teething:
   • excessive drooling
   • crying
   • mild irritability
   • increased finger sucking
   • desire to bite hard objects

3. Provide information on soothing techniques for teething:
   • Gently rub/massage gums with finger or cold washcloth.
   • Offer cold, refrigerated (not frozen) teething ring.
   • Give acetaminophen and/or topical anesthetic for persistent pain.

4. Inform parents that teething pain occurs as the tooth breaks through the periodontal membrane, with resulting inflammation. Once the tooth breaks through, teething pain diminishes.

5. Inform parents that fever over 100°F, diarrhea, and vomiting are not symptoms of teething.

6. Suggest parents call if they have questions or concerns.

$\mathcal{V}$OMITING

Nedra Skale, RN, MS, CNA

Vomiting, usually accompanied by nausea, is common in childhood. When limited in duration and amount, vomiting is of little concern. Inform parents that

1. Spitting up or dribbling of unswallowed formula from an infant's mouth is normal.
2. Regurgitation of undigested formula from the stomach sometimes occurs with burping.
3. Projectile vomiting, ejected with great force, from either an infant or a child is not normal. Projectile vomiting usually is not preceded by nausea.
4. If their child is vomiting, the parents need to note potential causes, frequency, severity, and if associated with coughing, pain, diarrhea, fever, headache, or changes in mental status.
5. Parents need to note content and color, if possible, to relate to physician.
6. The child's temperature should be measured and fever controlled.
7. Children with mild illness appear well, with no signs of infection or dehydration. Parents need to observe for any changes.
8. Children with moderate illness have signs of infection, systemic disease, weight loss or lack of weight gain, or prolonged vomiting. Parent should seek medical attention as soon as possible.
9. Children with severe illness are dehydrated, appear toxic, and may exhibit behavioral/mental status changes. Parent needs to seek medical attention immediately.
10. Offering the infant electrolyte solutions or Jello-water during acute illness will help prevent dehydration. If vomiting has not subsided in 24 hr, the infant should be evaluated for dehydration and further treatment. Breast-feeding does not need to be interrupted in most cases.
11. Children should be offered clear liquids during acute illness. Solid foods and thick liquids may aggravate nausea and vomiting.
12. A dietary/nutritional consult may be helpful if food intolerance is suspected.

13. Once infection (otitis) or systemic disease (flu) has resolved, the vomiting will stop.
14. See Gastroesophageal Reflux/Pyloric Stenosis, p 151.

REFERENCES: HEALTH TEACHING GUIDES

Barkin, R. & Rosen, P. (1990). *Emergency pediatrics: A guide to ambulatory care*, St. Louis, MO: C. V. Mosby Co.

Jones, N. E. (1993). Childhood residential injuries. *Maternal-Child Nursing Journal, 18*, 168–172.

Sheloo, S. (Ed.). (1991). *Caring for your baby and young child: Birth to age 5*. New York, NY: Bantam.

APPENDIX A: RESOURCES

American Academy of Pediatrics
141 Northwest Point Blvd.
P.O. Box 927
Elk Grove Village, IL 60009–0927

Association for the Care of Children's Health
7910 Woodmont Ave.
Suite 300
Bethesda, MD 20814
  1–301–654–6549

Asthma and Allergy Foundation of America
1125 15th Street, NW, Suite 502
Washington, DC, 20005

Child and Youth Services Administration
1120 19th St. N.W.
Suite 700
Washington DC 20036
  1–202–673–7783

Clearinghouse on Child Abuse and Neglect
P.O. Box 1182
Washington, DC 20013

Juvenile Diabetes Foundation International
432 Park Avenue South
New York, NY 10016
  1–212–889–7575
  1–800–223–1138

Medic-Alert Foundation International
2323 Colorado Ave.
Turlock, CA 95380
    1–800–ID-ALERT

Midwest Association for Sickle Cell Anemia
185 N. Wabash Ave.
Suite 1600
Chicago, IL 60601
    1–312–663–5700

National Institute of Child Health and Human Development
Building 31 Room 2A-32
9000 Rockville Pike
Bethesda, MD 20892
    1–301–496–5133

National Pediculosis Association
P.O. Box 149
Newton, MA 02169
    1–800–446–4NPA

The American Dietetic Association
216 W. Jackson Boulevard
Chicago, IL 60606-6995
    1–312–899–0040
    1–800–877–1600

U.S. Department of Health and Human Services
Public Health Service
Centers for Disease Control
Atlanta, GA 30333

INDEX

Note: Page numbers followed by t indicate tables; numbers followed by f indicate figures.